The Lomidine Files

The Lomidine Files

The Untold Story of a Medical Disaster in Colonial Africa

Guillaume Lachenal

Translated by Noémi Tousignant

Johns Hopkins University Press   *Baltimore*

Originally published as *Le médicament qui devait sauver l'Afrique. Un scandale pharmaceutique aux colonies*

© Éditions La Découverte, Paris, France, 2014
Translation © Johns Hopkins University Press, 2017
All rights reserved. Published 2017
Printed in the United States of America on acid-free paper
9 8 7 6 5 4 3 2 1

Johns Hopkins University Press
2715 North Charles Street
Baltimore, Maryland 21218-4363
www.press.jhu.edu

Library of Congress Cataloging-in-Publication Data

Names: Lachenal, Guillaume, 1978–, author.
Title: The Lomidine files: the untold story of a medical disaster in colonial Africa / Guillaume Lachenal; translated by Noémi Tousignant.
Other titles: Médicament qui devait sauver l'Afrique. English | Lomidine scandal and treating sleeping sickness in Africa
Description: Baltimore: Johns Hopkins University Press, 2017. | Translation of: Le médicament qui devait sauver l'Afrique : un scandale pharmaceutique aux colonies / Guillaume Lachenal. Paris : La Découverte, 2014. | Includes bibliographical references and index.
Identifiers: LCCN 2016051704| ISBN 9781421423234 (hardcover : alk. paper) | ISBN 9781421423241 (electronic) | ISBN 1421423235 (hardcover : alk. paper) | ISBN 1421423243 (electronic)
Subjects: | MESH: Trypanosomiasis, African—drug therapy | Pentamidine—adverse effects | Colonialism—history | Ethics, Medical—history | History, 20th Century | Africa | France
Classification: LCC RA644.T69 | NLM WC 705 | DDC 614.5/33—dc23
LC record available at https://lccn.loc.gov/2016051704

A catalog record for this book is available from the British Library.

Special discounts are available for bulk purchases of this book. For more information, please contact Special Sales at 410-516-6936 or specialsales@press.jhu.edu.

Johns Hopkins University Press uses environmentally friendly book materials, including recycled text paper that is composed of at least 30 percent post-consumer waste, whenever possible.

Contents

The Lomidine Files

An Anthropology of Colonial Unreason

In the early morning of November 12, 1954, the Service d'hygiène mobile et de prophylaxie (Mobile Hygiene and Prophylaxis Service) made its annual stop in Gribi, a village in eastern Cameroon. All the villagers, women and children included, gathered, as they did every year, for their injection of Lomidine. The preventive administration of Lomidine to entire populations, then called "total Lomidinization," was a priority and a source of pride for the postwar colonial health services. The technique's efficacy was unprecedented: a single injection of Lomidine conferred protection for several months against infection by trypanosomes, the parasites that cause sleeping sickness. In the face of an epidemic disease considered to be the main obstacle to demographic growth and to the project of *mise en valeur*[1] in the African colonies, this new strategy kindled great hope. Now, for the first time, eradication was within reach. Indeed, no new cases of the disease had been reported in the Gribi area in 1954.

The team worked efficiently. In just two days, four nurses surveyed, examined, and Lomidinized more than a thousand individuals. On the evening of November 13, a "European health assistant" by the name of Ansellem left Gribi to spend the night in the nearby regional capital of Yokadouma, 30 kilometers away.

An unexpected event interrupted his evening rest: a truck arrived carrying a resident of Gribi who complained of a painful abscess in the buttocks, which appeared to have resulted from the Lomidine injection. Ansellem did not seem worried by the incident and kept to the plan for the tour. The following morning, his team Lomidinized another three hundred people in a neighboring village. Later that day, however, the news from Gribi was alarming: three individuals had died, and another dozen, all Lomidinized two days earlier, had developed worrisome abscesses. During the evening, a truck arrived: its twenty-one passengers were in critical condition. Their buttocks and thighs were very swollen, and there were signs of putrefaction and bursting in their muscles; their "general state" was very "altered." During the night, two patients died. Four or five fell into a coma.

The death toll climbed by the hour. A catastrophe was looming, and the diagnosis was soon obvious: the shot of Lomidine had caused a bacterial infection that progressed to gas gangrene, spreading from the buttock to the rest of the body, leading to swelling and bursting in affected tissues. Despite the arrival of medical backup on November 15, the "accident of Yokadouma" resulted in a total of more than three hundred cases of gangrene and thirty-two deaths—one of the most violent medical catastrophes in African history.

This book is a biography of Lomidine. It traces this medicine's trajectory from its first trials during the Second World War, when it was introduced as a miracle cure for sleeping sickness, to its abandonment in the late 1950s, when a series of incidents in Gribi and elsewhere brought Lomidinization campaigns to a grinding halt. My broader aim, however, is more ambitious: by selecting as a historical object this white powder, a powder injected more than ten million times in Africa during the 1950s, I am experimenting with a novel form of inquiry into the relation between medicine and colonialism. Considering this drug as a therapeutic agent, a technology of government, a commodity as well as an object of expertise, belief, storytelling, and controversy and by tracking its history as it unfolded, I seek to study medicine as a tool of colonial power and as the stage of its legitimation—and its contestation. Inverting this relation, I seek in addition to understand the imperial dimension of the biomedical revolution of the second half of the twentieth century.

Lomidine's history opens a window onto the daily life of the colonial "modernization" program implemented after World War II, revealing its underside: its racial logics, coercive apparatus, and constitutive inefficacy along with the unreason inherent in its characteristic principles of rationality, authority, and evidence—what I call their *bêtise* (this term is discussed in more detail below). From sanitary utopia to health catastrophe, the history of Lomidine lays bare the messianic, mediocre, enthusiastic, and obstinate contribution of medicine to European imperialism. It allows for a reexamination of the colonial dream of an Africa liberated from disease and of the hopes and lives left in its wake.

An Awkward Ruin

I will start this story where it ends: in the late 2000s in eastern France, on the bank of the Doubs in the middle of the industrial wasteland of the Rhodi-

acéta factory—known to the locals as "la Rhodia." During the Trente Glorieuses (Glorious Thirty),[2] Rhodia was among the landmark textile factories of
Rhône-Poulenc, then the biggest chemical and pharmaceutical firm in France.
With more than three thousand workers producing nylon and other synthetic
fibers in the 1960s, the factory was the region's industrial pride and glory and
an exemplary site of French-style Fordism—as well as of its contestation in
1967–68. Hit hard by the oil crisis and by the ensuing corporate restructuring,
the factory closed its doors in the early 1980s, after several business plans and
as many promises of recovery and revitalization.[3] All that is left of Rhodia's
glorious past in Besançon is a huge, cumbersome ruin, too much trouble to
destroy and too expensive to restore.

A single functional building remains. It houses the Société d'archivage moderne (Society for Modern Archiving; SAM), a company specializing in "the
stocking, conservation and destruction of archives," according to its website.[4]
Created when Rhodia closed, the SAM now employs about twenty workers,
several of whom were reclassified from jobs in the former factory; the archivist
who received me, for example, was formerly a Tergal spinner. Thus, all that
is left of Rhodia is a modest archiving company; it is as if the act of archiving
this history operates as both a continuation and a parody of factory work. The
SAM inherited part of the archives of the Rhône-Poulenc corporation, which
became Aventis, then Sanofi, after a series of mergers, dissolutions, and acqui-
sitions. Among these archives I found three precious boxes: they contained
the only files I could access on Lomidine from its former manufacturer, then
one of the world's biggest pharmaceutical firms.

The files came from the Usines du Rhône (Rhône Factories) in Saint-Fons
near Lyons, where Lomidine powder was processed and packaged. They record
a thousand minutely detailed debates about the best ways of filling, stopper-
ing, labeling, wrapping, storing, and shipping, mainly to Africa, flasks and
ampules of Lomidine. These are tedious questions that no one, not even specialists, are interested in today. But they were questions of life or death, as we
will see, on a November day in 1954 in Gribi, eastern Cameroon.

I begin this book with these archives, even though I read them—after several years spent looking for and then gaining access to them—at the very end
of my investigation. Because of their content, form, and current status, these
archives allow me to articulate some of the fundamental ideas underlying my
project. They speak, above all, of material matters—of the smell and texture of
a powder, its dust and impurities, of the aesthetics of a label and the fragility

of a flask. These issues lie at the heart of my inquiry: to proceed by way of materiality is, for me, a research strategy that allows for the circumvention of the "historiographical cliché" of an encounter between colonizer and colonized,[5] and this strategy allows me to locate myself beyond texts and the language of colonial experts. These archives also reveal a need to think of colonial medicine in Africa beyond the borders of each European empire: the collected correspondence traces a transnational and inter-imperial network, connecting the secretariat of one of France's biggest chemical factories with Portuguese Angola, the Belgian Congo, and French Guinea via Vitry-sur-Seine, Léopoldville, and Liverpool; this network was simultaneously commercial, medical, and scientific. Finally, these archives speak of the passage of time, of what lasts and of what vanishes beyond political history's major watersheds. With its gutted walls, old machines, and factory workers turned into archivists, the Rhodia wasteland is a ruin of modernity that both describes and parodies the hopes and projects of France's era of modernization. More unexpectedly, the Lomidine files kept, somewhat accidentally, in the last of its buildings also make Rhodia an improbable remnant of empire, which sets the Trente Glorieuses of French science and industry against their imperial and African backdrop.[6]

Biography of Debris

Like Rhodia, Lomidine is a troublesome ruin, debris of empire. Lomidine (also known by the name of Pentamidine) is a surprising, but not necessarily an exceptional, case in medical history.[7] Throughout the 1950s, it was seen as a miracle drug, an emblem of "modern medicine" in Africa, and it was administered preventively and compulsorily to entire regions. Beginning in the late 1960s, however, its status radically changed. After two decades of mass campaigns punctuated by horrific therapeutic accidents, a series of laboratory experiments completely revised the state of knowledge on the drug's efficacy and safety—and even its mode of action. A consensus was reached, which remains undisputed: Lomidine has no preventive effects. It does not protect (or at least not very well, certainly not for several months) healthy individuals, and it exposes those individuals to unacceptable risks, particularly for the heart. This does not imply that Lomidinization campaigns played no role in arresting the epidemic progression of sleeping sickness; the drug did, apparently, contribute to the interruption of transmission at the population level—though this is not how its mechanism was understood at the time. Yet as the

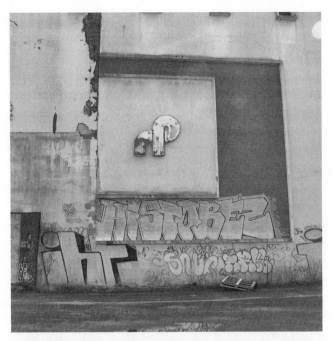

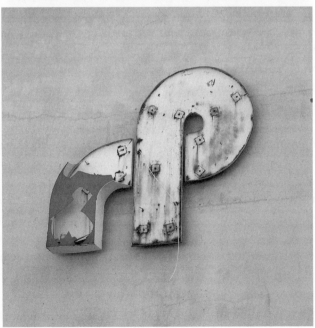

Rhodia wasteland, Besançon, 2008. Photos by author.

prospect of eradication definitively receded, preventive Lomidine came to be seen as a "pointless, dangerous, and thus pointlessly dangerous" technique, in the words of French doctor René Labusquière, one of the major postwar figures of the colonial medical corps.[8] After such a reversal, the moment of glory of "total Lomidinization" has become difficult to comprehend and even to narrate, which may explain why historians have remained so silent about it. Lomidinization, which was erected as a monument to the colonial health enterprise in the 1950s, had to then be erased from official histories of tropical medicine. What remains are carefully archived shelves full of publicity brochures, reports, correspondence, medical theses, conference proceedings, and field manuals describing Lomidinization campaigns. The wonder drug has become embarrassing: too awkward for the hagiographers and too technical or anecdotal for critical historical narratives.

Retrospectively, Lomidinization appears to be a technique that worked but for the "wrong" reasons; the therapeutic rationale, to borrow current terminology, has revealed itself to be a public health strategy based on mere faith. By giving away the denouement of the plot from the outset, my goal is not to expose colonial doctors as having operated under an illusion, as having been mistaken about Lomidine, and thus to write what Bachelard called a "judged history."[9] I seek instead to make heuristic use of the retrospective judgment on Lomidine. How is it possible to understand its obvious success, doctors' enthusiasm for it, and its routine use in mass campaigns, when we now know that Lomidine is an extremely tricky drug to handle, that it does not work preventively, and that it is very painful when injected—an example of what French clinicians call a *cochonnerie*: a nasty, difficult, yet indispensable drug?[10] This question might be accused of anachronism: historians, in such situations, often opt for the pretense of being unaware of "what we now know" in order to avoid writing history backward.[11] Yet at the risk of shocking, the end of the story guides my inquiry because it spurs attentiveness—perhaps a bit more than usual—to the (in)efficacy of the drug itself as an unstable, material substance; to its prodigious successes and its misfires; to its agency; and to how this agency destabilized or reassured the drug's proponents, or left them indifferent.[12]

This approach places the incoherence of daily practice at the center of an inquiry on the processes that afforded coherence and strength to colonial medical power. How did colonial experts understand and resolve—by sometimes violent means—the uncertainties and fragility of their own techniques and programs? What world views, what technical and scientific calculations, what ethical and political choices allowed—even as contradictions, problems, and resistance arose—for the determined and enthusiastic implementation of Lomidinization, which indeed grew even more determined and enthusiastic *as* contradictions, problematic incidents, and resistance arose? To put it more crudely: How did it become possible and acceptable for thirty-two people to die in Gribi, near Yokadouma, on a single day in November 1954 after they were injected with a medicine that was already (half-)known to not really protect against a disease that, in any case, was no longer present in the area? My project is thus both a biography of a technoscientific object and a historical anthropology of colonial unreason.

Lomidine and the "Colonial Disease"

The biography of Lomidine sheds light on a relatively unknown but crucial phase in the colonial control of sleeping sickness—an epidemic that has played a major role in African history. Sleeping sickness (African human trypanosomiasis) is a parasitic infection caused by a trypanosome and transmitted by the tsetse fly (glossina);[13] it is prevalent in intertropical Africa in a band that stretches from Senegal to Lake Victoria. Its common name refers to the neurological and psychiatric symptoms associated with the advanced stages of the disease. Sleeping sickness was defined as a health priority by the colonial states of Central Africa in the first years of the twentieth century. At that time, the disease, then of unknown etiology, grew to epidemic proportions, particularly in the Great Lakes region and the Congo Basin. This unprecedented outbreak was both a symptom and a result of the social, ecological, and demographic crisis caused by colonial conquest in this region; classic estimates suggest that Central Africa lost half of its population between 1880 and 1910.[14]

Mobilization against this epidemic stimulated the birth and institutionalization of "tropical medicine" as a discipline in both Europe and the colonial world. A series of expeditions and study missions was organized, both in collaboration and in competition, by a loose set of semi-public institutions, such as the Institut Pasteur (Pasteur Institute) and the Liverpool School of Tropical Medicine, and by scientific societies, colonial lobbyists, eminent scientists such as the German Robert Koch, and private individuals like King Leopold. Their findings provided a basis for determining the etiological and clinical profile of the disease.[15] In just a few years, between 1902 and 1907, researchers managed to identify the disease's parasite, vector, and animal reservoir and to describe its course in humans, beginning with a first stage lasting up to several years during which few perceptible symptoms appear, then progressing, with highly variable speed and intensity from one individual to another, to a more severe, eventually fatal affliction. The microbe hunt led by European scientists and the ensuing initial therapeutic successes were given a high public profile. The tsetse fly thus became a familiar figure of colonial propaganda; along with the image of the pith-helmeted doctor hunched over a microscope, it made its way into the textbooks of metropolitan schoolchildren.[16]

Historians have displayed great interest in the large-scale sleeping sickness control programs deployed from Upper Volta to Tanganyika during the interwar period.[17] These programs varied in form, over time, and according to context, alternately targeting the tsetse fly, animal reservoirs, population movements, or the parasite itself through chemotherapy. Yet they all shared a particularly ambitious conception of public health, relying on a centralized, coercive, and militarized apparatus. In some rural areas, sleeping sickness interventions were the main expression of the colonial state; they also inspired the pursuit of sanitary utopias, in which medical action took on the features of a social engineering project.[18] By mobilizing hundreds of doctors and thousands of African auxiliaries across European empires, the control of sleeping sickness also catalyzed the emergence of an imperial medical profession—called *la trypano* in francophone areas—and the creation of a specific professional corps, with its own rituals and heroes, such as Eugène Jamot.[19]

The populations of affected zones were summoned to compulsory sessions of diagnostic screening and treatment, particularly in the Belgian Congo, Cameroon, Afrique occidentale française (French West Africa; AOF), and Afrique équatoriale française (French Equatorial Africa; AEF). These mass campaigns were experiments with an innovative form of standardized collective medicine; they had, at the time, no equivalents in the imperial metropoles in France or Belgium. If the epidemic itself, triggered by the "scramble for Africa" of the late nineteenth century, was in a way the colonial disease par excellence, the campaigns launched to control it similarly constituted an archetype of colonial medicine. They were a mode of medical practice that prescribed colonial order as much as they were produced by it.[20] By making the management of the population—as both biological entity and human capital—their objective and horizon, these campaigns engaged in a pure form of biopolitics, as defined by Michel Foucault. Their ambition and logics anticipated (and in some cases directly contributed to) the racial turn in European biopolitics of the 1930s and 1940s.[21]

The control of sleeping sickness was photogenic and spectacular; it later became a topic of prolific memorial production, proffering figures and stories to both revisionist and apologist historians of the "colonial enterprise"; Niall Ferguson, for example, used (inaccurately captioned) photos of Dr. Jamot in his "TED Talk."[22] This battle against disease was not only a fascinating feature of imperial cultures, it is also embedded in the genealogy of contemporary humanitarianism. During the sleeping sickness campaigns, photos on glossy paper of gaunt African children circulated for the first time—such images would have a long shelf life in the European media—while the laid-back yet sophisticated figure of the French doctor, fighting an ever-losing battle against disease, African ignorance, and Western bureaucracy, also made his first appearance.[23]

Lomidine has been a forgotten player in all this. Histories of sleeping sickness generally focus on the monumental actors of the interwar era, with the period after 1945 tacked on as an epilogue. Chronicles of medical progress do note that Lomidine revitalized an aging therapeutic arsenical, which, until the 1940s, was limited to rather toxic, arsenic-based trypanocide molecules. Yet the radical novelty of its preventive use (what is now called chemoprophylaxis) is rarely pointed out. Lomidinization "accidents," the accepted euphemism at the time, are known today by only a handful of tropical medicine specialists.[24]

This omission is especially surprising given that Lomidinization and its "accidents" happened during sleeping sickness control's moment of triumph, at a time when imminent eradication was announced on a regular basis. This was also a time of new problems, however, as the liberalization of colonial regimes recast authoritarian modes of population management as an increasingly sensitive issue. The 1950s were a golden age for colonial medicine, which was bolstered by unprecedented technical means and political will; yet the '50s were also a decade of tensions and violence in French colonies as well as in Belgian, British, and Portuguese Africa. Never before had colonial sanitary utopianism been pushed further in its logic and contradictions. The biography of Lomidine is a narrative thread with which to grasp late colonialism as a moment of both reform and reaction, when racial hierarchies were simultaneously undermined and reaffirmed.

The Empire of *Bêtise*

Historians often describe colonial medicine as an instrument for the rational ordering of the colonized world, imposing its hierarchies, values, and identities onto people and things. Colonial medicine, which became a scientific discipline of its own, did indeed serve as an ideology and tool of empire: by embodying the *mission civilisatrice* (civilizing mission), by facilitating military conquest, and by protecting the health of colonists. It was also a strategic site of intervention into colonized societies, a form of government of bodies and populations that, in its reach, far exceeded the goal of controlling disease. In the field of medicine, the colonies were even considered in situ laboratories, sites for the testing of therapeutic, urbanist, and bureaucratic techniques to be reimported to the metropole.[25]

Yet the case of Lomidine does not fully align with this critical, Foucault-inspired reading.[26] There are several reasons such a reading would be incomplete. First, there was, as historians such as Fred Cooper remind us, a gulf between colonial intentions and realizations, and the great biopolitical projects often got mired in the lack of means and the internal tensions of colonial states.[27] Above all, such an analysis, by taking doctors at their words, would completely miss what Achille Mbembe describes as the "contribution of 'misfires,' of the unexpected and of 'disorder'," which were at the heart of the colonial disciplinary project; this dimension, he points out, "has until now been reconstructed with an impressive lack of precision."[28]

Lomidine opens up an approach to colonial history that takes a "misfire" as its point of departure; its history is that of a mediocre medicine, which would fail even to provoke scandal. Lomidine was a drug that did not really work—or, to put it a bit differently, that worked a little, but not for the right reasons. It is precisely because Lomidine could not protect individuals per se that it was prescribed for application to entire regions until it became a medicine "for the race," one that was evaluated and administered—if needed, by force—exclusively on a collective scale. Its misfires were obvious to doctors, but they were also galvanizing. To account for this episode, it is difficult to rely on the categories usually mobilized by historians, who are inclined to speak of the colonies as an ordered world, dominated by reason and colonial law, or to describe colonial doctors, in the manner of Bruno Latour and of science studies, as archetypal embodiments of the scientist-entrepreneur, at once producers of knowledge and reformers of society.[29] The minor history of Lomidine introduces disorder and doubt into such grand narratives: it poses the question of how to characterize what looks, retrospectively, like a colossal failure, which was promoted in real time with an arrogance that seems difficult to take seriously today.

The case of Lomidine invites another way of telling the history of science and of colonial medicine. The idea is not only to keep pointing out—against a somewhat naïve, or fascinated, reading of biopolitical projects—the thousand contradictions and setbacks of colonial modernization but also to reexamine what has been left out of the historical field of vision: the constitutive powerlessness, hubris, and irrationality of colonial government. The existing gap in historiographical thinking is particularly puzzling considering that the rational dimension of colonial policies was systematically criticized from the very start: colonists themselves mocked the "life-size experiments" (one of doctors' favorite phrases), "pilot projects," and other ambitious undertakings of colonial *mise en valeur*, not to mention their perplexed and incredulous interpretation by colonized subjects.[30] Literature has been particularly inclined to critiques of colonial and scientific megalomania, echoing broader judgments about experimental medicine, including colonial medicine.[31] Surprisingly, this often humorous and sometimes despairing reflexive dimension of colonial modernity has been completely neglected by scholars, who seem to be the only ones left who believe in colonial doctors' demiurgic power to discipline bodies and order the world.[32]

In this book, I launch an inquiry into the negatives that worked within colonial logic, which made it "a reason that was at once religious, mystical, messianic, military and utopian," as Mbembe puts it.[33] The goal is not to stage a romantic confrontation between "other" systems of thought and action and "Western rationality," embodied in the imposition of grids on indigenous spaces and societies. Rather, I seek to give an account of the "double structure of ignorance and impotence" in which the colonial will to know and to intervene was embedded.[34] There are several possible ways of turning on its head the description of an omniscient, omnipotent, and rational colonial power. One is to reexamine the way in which it cultivated ignorance,[35] even madness, to "move," as Johannes Fabian proposes, "the critique of colonialism from questions of guilt to questions of error."[36] Another is to attend, as Warwick Anderson and Nancy Hunt do, to how the "nerves" of colonial agents,[37] especially doctors, were harshly tested, to the extent of stimulating the emergence of a specialized medicopsychiatric infrastructure—and publishing industry—in both colonies and metropoles.[38] As Fabian shows in his counterhistory of late nineteenth-century Africanist ethnology, the colonial operation of ordering the African continent was often carried out by scientists who were exhausted, intoxicated, and knocked out by fever, whose ways of knowing deviated, to put it mildly, from cold rationality.[39] This body of work suggests that the colonial knowledge regime was anchored as much in a culture of ignorance and inaction as it was in the quest for order and scientific facts that historians have so prolifically written about.

In this book, I am interested in yet another pathology of reason, one described by Gustave Flaubert, Gilles Deleuze, and Roland Barthes using the French term *bêtise*. The history of Lomidinization and its daily catastrophes cannot be reduced to the story of a medical error, an ethical infraction, or a mad experiment; rather, it must be the story of a technique that *was* scientific and that produced effects that were both dramatically uncertain and taken into account *as such*. How is it possible to understand the persistent determination, even as the number of incidents grew, to use the drug to the very end without assuming that doctors were either cynical, blind, or demented? This question pushes us to attend to the rational calculations and subjective dispositions that were necessary for Lomidine to be used on a massive scale and to their underlying and validating hypotheses. It points to the problem of an *active* production of trust in the medicine. It brings us to a series of questions that I borrow from Ann Stoler: "How much [did] the conditions of Empire produce stupefied serene states as well as racial anxieties, or something that uneasily combine[d] ways of not knowing and obliquely knowing at the same time?"[40] Which affective and cognitive dispositions secured belief in the effectiveness of the technique and in the necessity of eradication? How was the confidence of ordinary colonial doctors generated and maintained? How were the failures of the technique interpreted and resolved, so that its use was resumed in an even more joyous manner—comparable to the case of Bouvard and Pécuchet going from experiment to experiment in the eponymous novel by Flaubert? What forms of "knowledge and/or of disinhibiting ignorance," to take up Jean-Baptiste Fressoz's analysis,[41] allowed and organized the repetition of catastrophes such as those of Gribi? What lifestyles, what rhetorical and technical apparatus, what scientific and lay representations—of race, of Africans, of science, of empire, of the future—defined the postwar version of colonialism, which was, as Fred Cooper writes, "at its most reformist, its most interventionist, its most arrogantly assertive?"[42] In short, what remains surprising and needs to be understood in the doctors' eradicating project of the 1950s is the unshakable trust that pervaded it despite a context of profound uncertainty and insecurity. This serenity, which would envelop the dead of Gribi with silence and certainty in November 1954, is what I suggest is best captured by the term "bêtise."

Bêtise is reason at its most arrogantly assertive. As many have noted, including Avital Ronell, Jacques Derrida, and Isabelle Stengers, the term is untranslatable.[43] It is usually rendered as "stupidity," but as Stengers emphasizes, "this is not unproblematic—stupidity invokes *stupor*, sleep, while 'la bêtise' . . . has nothing passive about it."[44] I see bêtise as a particular species of unreason, radically distinct from error: an enthusiastic and enterprising form of stupidity, a confident and calculated form of foolishness; "pig-headedness" is perhaps the closest English equivalent (although bêtise is a human privilege). Thus, the specific sense in which I use it does not refer to a deficiency, but rather to an intrinsic potential within reason. It manifests when reason, anchored in its evidence base and in logical, scientific procedures, gains a mineral and monumental confidence—it "takes the nature of granite," says Flaubert. It is an excessive, active, confident, determined—unshakable—deployment of reason; it is, in other words, a form of *déraison* (unreason) that is not only a lack but an extension of reason, as suggested by the French language, where the prefix *dé-* can refer, ambiguously, to both deficiency and enhancement.[45] In its purest form, the concept is a tautology, such as in the statement "after all, natives are natives," which a young Englishwoman says, with disarming logic and goodwill, in a colonial novel by George Orwell.[46] According to the definition given by the philosopher Alain Roger, it is endowed with the calm strength of good or common sense.

Although bêtise has been a topic of much reflection in the philosophical and literary fields, stemming in particular from its problematization by Flaubert and then by Deleuze and Barthes,[47] historians and anthropologists of science have avoided engaging with it. Jean-Marc Lévy-Leblond thus remarks that while the figure of madness is fairly well addressed by the scholarly and lay imagery of science, the "necessary and constitutive unreason of science—that blindness that follows its furrow without letting itself be distracted . . . the myopic determination of those who plough the glebe of the world with a more effective science" has been consistently overlooked, despite having inspired an extraordinary body of literary work.[48] The topic has been no more popular in colonial studies, even with all the attention given to "colonial madness" and to agnotology (study of the social production of ignorance),[49] nor among medical anthropologists, even though some have written chronicles of what might be called the "bloopers" of public health.[50] Paul Farmer has even made the issue of "stupid deaths" the point of departure of a radical critique of global inequalities in health.[51] The call of Isabelle Stengers to "name the stupidity," to "recount the manner in which stupidity has captured the scientific adventure, has contributed to putting the power of proof in the service of public order" has remained unanswered[52]—perhaps, I must add, for good reasons.

To diagnose others' stupidity, bêtise, or related forms of unreason is risky. That the accusation of stupidity was part of the colonial and medical universes of the nineteenth and twentieth centuries, and can thus be treated as a "value judgment in indirect speech," to follow Paul Veyne's analysis of the historiographical problem of foolishness,[53] is an acceptable but rather limited justification for its use by a historian. To name and to point out stupidity, even with irony, inevitably comes from a position of assumed superiority and thus plays dangerously with the limits of one's own intelligence. The problem is a familiar one; it stimulated the formal work done by Flaubert in *Bouvard et Pécuchet*, in which the enunciation of bêtise is made possible by the device of free indirect discourse, which creates and maintains permanent uncertainty as to who is speaking: the author, the characters themselves, the authors they cite and mimic, or the common sense of their times.[54] In other words, this particular form of unreason is expressible only in the absence of a voice that can name it from the outside and that finds itself thus excluded. Stupidity (in another person) thus creates a writing challenge that perhaps only a text made into pure description, into an encyclopedia entry, or into a collage can surmount—by putting on hold what Roland Barthes calls the "metalanguage" of irony.[55]

I cannot hope to fully succeed, but I still find it worthwhile to underline the heuristic potential of the notion. It shines light from a new angle onto colonial medicine's will to eradicate—its will to conclude, to stick with the Flaubertian definition of bêtise. Bêtise makes it possible to take seriously the enthusiasm of colonial medicine's actors, who would later call themselves "boy scouts of public health";[56] it gives a name to their political thought, which was at once euphoric and aggressive, racialized and universalist, and which was one of the foundations of late colonialism's development programs. Finally, naming stupidity or bêtise has a critical and an ethical function: unlike madness, the term is not a distancing or an othering device; following Anne Herschberg-Pierrot's expression, the "empire of bêtise" is universal and inclusive. To name the unreason specific to the episodes described in this book is not to lock it up in a colonial museum of horrors, but rather to bring it closer to us by allowing it to resonate in the present. This is the only condition under which this history can formulate its critique: my book is not addressed to a handful of forgotten colonial doctors, but to the serene entrepreneurs of contemporary global

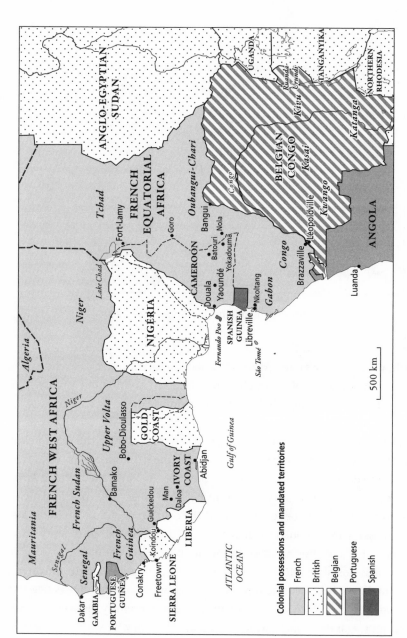

West and Central Africa circa 1940

Colonial possessions and mandated territories

French
British
Belgian
Portuguese
Spanish

500 km

ATLANTIC OCEAN

Mauritania

FRENCH WEST AFRICA

Algeria

Senegal

Dakar

GAMBIA

PORTUGUESE GUINEA

French Guinea

Conakry

Freetown

SIERRA LEONE

LIBERIA

Koindou

Guéckedou

Man

Daloa

IVORY COAST

Abidjan

Bamako

French Sudan

Upper Volta

Bobo-Dioulasso

GOLD COAST

Gulf of Guinea

Niger

Niger

Lake Chad

Tchad

Fort-Lamy

NIGERIA

FRENCH EQUATORIAL AFRICA

CAMEROON

Douala

Yaoundé

Goro

Batouri

Yokadouma

Nola

Bangui

Oubangui-Chari

ANGLO-EGYPTIAN SUDAN

UGANDA

BELGIAN CONGO

Ruanda-Urundi

Kivu

Kasai

Katanga

TANGANYIKA

NORTHERN RHODESIA

Congo

Kwango

Léopoldville

Brazzaville

Congo

Gabon

Nkoltang

Libreville

SPANISH GUINEA

Fernando Poo

São Tomé

ANGOLA

Luanda

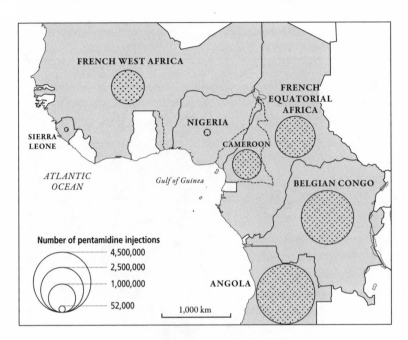

Number of pentamidine injections, 1944–1960

health, who are busy saving Africa with "simple solutions." It is to those who consider, in the words of Teju Cole, "the world [as] nothing but a problem to be solved by enthusiasm," that this book is addressed.[57]

The history of Lomidine is not a representative one: during the same period in Africa there were less embarrassing episodes, medicines that worked as they should, and doctors who saved lives. Furthermore, colonial medicine in Africa was for the most part a story of African health workers and African patients who, potentially, could bend and subvert the colonizers' rules. This book does not address them. Colonial medicine was, at times, an extraordinarily effective apparatus and thus an object of desire; it is not uncommon in Africa to come across nostalgic references to the time of big public health campaigns. To highlight the minuscule and preoccupying history of Lomidine is selective and somewhat unfair to what was happening concurrently elsewhere. I take responsibility for this choice, which goes hand in hand with the narrative form of this book: telling a story is always, as Susan Sontag writes in one of her late publications, a "shrinking of the world."[58]

Lomidine is not among the great medicines of which biographies have been written, full of triumph and tragedy.[59] It has been a muted character, which fell far short of fulfilling its promise as a wonder drug yet remains useful in the treatment of several parasitic diseases, which are known, aptly, as "neglected diseases." It is a second-rate medicine, used mainly in the periphery of the Western world. Its successes and failures have not (or only marginally) been of concern to White people in Europe or the United States. Uncertain and prosaic, its biography is that of an injection that stings and dizzies, makes bodies vomit and piss, makes graphs fall and reports pile up, protects and kills.

Meet "Drug X"

It is a story that has never yet been written, the story of a drug so hush-hush that only the Colonial Office and half a dozen high-up experts know its name.

They hardly dare say so, but they hope it is going to lick a disease which kills millions of natives in the tropics every year—and hundreds of thousands of pounds' worth of cattle.

Why the secrecy?

There are people in Germany who could tell you that. For in 1921 Germany produced what was then the most promising weapon against sleeping sickness, a drug called Germanin. They refused to disclose the formula. But Germanin is only effective if you catch the disease in a very early stage.

Meanwhile . . . the disease is continually spreading. . . .

Four years ago the Colonial Office, stirring from its own brand of sleepiness, asked the Medical Research Council to tackle the problem. Dr. Lourie's visit to Gambia with Drug X (like most drugs still in the experimental stage, it is actually known by a number and not a name) is the result.

When Dr. Lourie, short and rather swarthy, arrives in the morning at his compounds in the jungle he finds fifty to 100 natives waiting for treatment. Some have walked there. Others have been carried. Dr. Lourie pricks the swollen glands in their necks and examines the fluid for trypanosomes, the deadly dragon-like parasites which cause the disease. Then he injects a dose of Drug X and tells them to come back in a week. For the undernourished native . . . the trypanosome is a deadly peril.

The extraordinary thing about this kind of research is that while it is highly organized and involves millions of careful tests, most of the best results are achieved by a colossal fluke. The search for Drug X is an example. Doctors know that the trypanosome lives on the sugar in the blood.

A Dr. von Jancso in Prague got the idea that if he gave the victim insulin, which reduced the blood-sugar, he could starve the trypanosomes. This was a completely crazy idea, because long before the trypanosomes felt hungry the patient would have died of insulin-shock. But the astonishing thing was that when he tried it, the patients got better. Or to be exact, they didn't [get better] when he used insulin, but they did when he used an artificial form of insulin made in Germany called synthalin.

Obviously it was the synthalin itself which was doing the trick. The danger is, the margin between a curative and a poisonous dose is very narrow.

At this point [researchers at] the Liverpool School of Tropical Medicine took up the battle. They proceeded to make all the other members of the synthalin family. From the synthalin family they progressed to neighbouring families and there one day they found, after cautious experiments, a drug which seemed to slay the trypanosomes without slaying the patient. The drug I have called Drug X. What is more, if you inject it into a healthy man, it seems to confer immunity to the disease.

Next year we shall learn the results. Perhaps the 40-year battle will have been won.

Gordon Taylor, "Meet Drug X," *Daily Express*, London, July 27, 1939.

CHAPTER ONE

The Wonder Drug

The biography of pentamidine begins with the kind of serendipitous discovery in which historians of medicine delight.[1]

In 1935, Nikolas von Jancso, a chemist at the University of Szeged in Hungary (who worked with his wife, Hertha, but she rarely makes it into historical accounts), embarked on a new path of inquiry into the value of substances causing hypoglycemia (low blood sugar) as sleeping sickness therapies. This was a reasonable premise, and the von Jancsos were respected researchers who collaborated with top German institutions.[2] Indeed, it had been known for decades that trypanosomes were avid consumers of glucose (the sugar in blood) both in vivo and in vitro. Postulating that a sudden drop in blood sugar in the host could kill off trypanosomes, the von Jancsos tested synthalin, a synthetic insulin substitute used to treat diabetes by lowering blood sugar levels. They successfully cured trypanosome-infected mice.[3]

News of the finding made its way to Professor Warrington Yorke, one of the major figures of British tropical medicine and holder of the Alfred Jones Chair of Tropical Medicine, the most prestigious position at one of the field's top institutions, the Liverpool School of Tropical Medicine.[4] Yorke specialized in pharmacological research, and the experimental study of trypanosomiasis was one of his areas of expertise. With Emanuel Lourie, a young researcher in his laboratory, Yorke immediately began testing synthalin in trypanosome-infected guinea pigs. Their results confirmed the effect found by the von Jancsos.[5] Unlike the Hungarian scientists, however, Yorke and Lourie demonstrated, by showing that synthalin worked at very low concentrations in vitro, that it acted directly on the parasite rather than via the hosts' metabolism (by depriving it of glucose). This meant that a new powerful trypanocide had been identified. One of their collaborators, a chemist from the National Institute for Medical Research in London, Dr. Harold King, then got to work synthesizing a series of compounds similar to synthalin. Among these, a few were powerful enough to fully cure test animals while being much less toxic than synthalin. In late 1937 King, Lourie, and Yorke announced in the *Lancet*, one of Britain's leading medical journals, the discovery of a new family of trypanocidal substances, the diamidines, which were unlike any existing compound for sleeping sickness treatment.[6] One of these diamidines would later be called pentamidine. The initial hypothesis turned out to be completely wrong, but the end result would have historians proclaiming that "lady luck" had struck again.[7]

A Colonial Wonder Drug

Along with sulfa drugs and penicillin, pentamidine was among a set of extraordinarily effective antimicrobial drugs developed in Europe over the span of less than a decade (1935–44). These wonder drugs, as they were then called, launched a "therapeutic revolution" that stemmed from unprecedentedly close connections among biological research, public health, industrial innovation, and mass consumption.[8] While this phenomenon has been well studied by historians,[9] the lesser-known history of pentamidine adds a revelation: the African colonies were not merely its backdrop. Peripheries of empire were laboratories of modernity for the emergence of biomedicine.

Africa was at the heart of the emergence of chemotherapy from the early years of the twentieth century;[10] indeed, the foundational work of the German scientist Paul Ehrlich, the inventor of the first magic bullet for syphilis (compound 606, or Salvarsan), began with the study of trypanosomiasis.[11] Pharmaceutical firms played their cards well by giving pride of place to their colonial contributions in public relations materials. New sleeping sickness drugs were widely publicized in interwar Europe. They became objects of nationalist competition; the best-known example is Germanin, a derivative of aniline launched by Bayer in 1925, which was displayed in German pro-imperial, then Nazi, propaganda. In France, Spécia (Société parisienne d'expansion chimique)—the pharmaceutical branch of the Rhône-Poulenc firm, the pride and glory of the French chemical industry—produced a famous film on the Mission Jamot that was presented at the Colonial Exhibition of 1931. We owe part of the visual archive of sleeping sickness control to the photographs commissioned by the firm in Congo and Cameroon.[12] At that time, trypanosomiasis was the polar opposite of a "neglected disease."

During the interwar period, companies began to address colonized societies as markets for their products. As objects of desire, fear, and trafficking in African societies, the miracle drugs manufactured by European industry acquired cultural significance; this was especially true for injectable treatments for syphilis, which provoked the ire of missionaries, who blamed them for making "the natives" nonchalant about venereal disease.[13] In short, it would be anachronistic to characterize as marginal the space in which the history of pentamidine would unfold.

Code Name: MB 800

Organized and funded by an alliance between the state and the pharmaceutical industry, the British discovery of pentamidine bears the imprint of big science. In late 1936, the Medical Research Council (MRC), an agency funded by medical insurance, launched a program to reestablish the vanguard position of British tropical medicine in the name of national prestige, supporting industry, and imperial development.[14] The program was supervised by Sir Henry Dale, a patron of British pharmacology in the interwar period, who had recently been awarded the Nobel Prize in medicine. He stimulated chemotherapy research on a national scale by granting scholarships and other forms of funding. The goal was to close the gap with Germany, where Germanin had just been launched by the Bayer firm as a miracle cure for trypanosomiasis.[15] Yorke's team at the Liverpool School of Tropical Medicine was among the main beneficiaries of this governmental funding agency, which covered the salary of two researchers, one of whom was Lourie.

Kept up to date on synthalin results from Liverpool, Henry Dale played the role of intermediary; to obtain new compounds, he contacted Harold King and Arthur Ewins, a chemist at May & Baker, one of the leading British pharmaceutical firms. The three men knew each other well—in British chemotherapy circles at the time, the boundary between public and private was "blurred"[16]— and thus it was a "colleague,"[17] as Dale put it, who took up the task of synthesizing a series of diamidine compounds in the May & Baker laboratories at Dagenham in East London. Of about thirty derivatives tested in mice, three stood out: stilbamidine, propamidine, and pentamidine, designated, as was customary, by their respective serial numbers, MB 744, MB 782, and MB 800.[18]

Over the following three-month period, the channels connecting May & Baker, the Liverpool School, and the MRC were busy. May & Baker provided compounds along with grant money to Yorke in Liverpool in exchange for priority access to his test results and a guaranteed right to file patents prior to publication.[19] Diamidines were tested in animal models of various parasitic infections, setting off an avalanche of articles in the *Annals of Tropical Medicine and Parasi-*

tology, the journal published by the school.[20] Diamidines sealed the alliance between the London-based firm and the Liverpool School, which would continue to provide the school with a reliable source of revenue into the late 1950s.[21]

If this arrangement—today we would call it by the dull name of "public-private partnership"—owed much to the personal connection between Yorke and Ewins, it was also congruent with the Liverpool School's long-standing strategy of obtaining financial support from Liverpool's major business actors. The best known was the shipping magnate and self-made man Alfred Jones, who saw tropical medicine as a tool that could contribute to the expansion of commerce with West Africa.[22] This arrangement was further facilitated by Warrington Yorke's own position as a businessman. Acting as a consultant and administrator for several firms, Yorke was also, since 1930, the head of his family's wire business, which made and sold mosquito screening for tropical houses.[23] Bolstered by private support, chemotherapy was showcased by the school, which planned to open a new building for it. As early as 1939, May & Baker was producing a considerable volume of all three diamidine compounds. Business and science were thriving.

Experiments and Patronage in the British Empire

Clinical trials, orchestrated by Warrington Yorke, were initiated even before the lab results were published. He solicited hospitals in Liverpool where seamen from around the British Empire were treated. "Syphilitics" who were "given" experimental malaria infections to treat states of general paralysis were thus cured of malaria.[24] A "Hindoo," who was "exceedingly ill" with kala azar, a parasitic disease caused by leishmania, was also saved.[25] As a patron of empire, Yorke arranged for samples of May & Baker's diamidines to be shipped to his correspondents and acquaintances, men who worked as colonial doctors in the Gambia, the Gold Coast, Nigeria, Sudan, Uganda, Palestine, and India, so they could be tested in hospitals and treatment campaigns. He then decided to send his assistant Emanuel Lourie to the Gambia to personally test the substances in humans.[26]

It was in Sierra Leone that the most ambitious experiments were conducted. The Liverpool School had a field station in Freetown—a small laboratory that it had staffed with a few scientists since 1922.[27] Warrington Yorke, who supervised the lab work from a distance, was informed in late April 1939 that an epidemic of sleeping sickness, a rare event in the colony at the time, had been signaled in the east near the borders with French Guinea and Liberia. Yorke seized the opportunity to offer his team's expertise to the colony's medical service. The Liverpool School, he wrote, "ought to offer to do a little more to help Sierra Leone in this sleeping sickness matter." He thus proposed to send Emanuel Lourie to the rescue.[28] On the verge of leaving for the Gambia, Lourie instead made his way to Sierra Leone to investigate the situation on the ground.

Fewer than fifteen days after boarding the *Accra* in Liverpool on May 31, loaded down with ampules of diamidines and journals for the laboratory's library, Lourie was already in the field in eastern Sierra Leone, near Koindu. He was accompanied by Thomas Davey, the director of the Freetown laboratory. Neither scientist had prior experience with trypanosomiasis: Lourie, who had until then made his name as a lab-based researcher, took his first steps in tropical Africa, while Davey confessed to Yorke that he had "no knowledge of the running of a sleeping sickness campaign."[29] To bring themselves up to speed, they contacted French doctors on the other side of the border who were old hands at running large-scale campaigns. Welcomed by their counterparts in Guéckédou, Guinea, the two men took part in one of the French team's treatment tours.[30] Back on "their" side of the border, they surveyed the affected areas to estimate the disease's prevalence. The numbers they reported were dramatic, with more than 25 percent of the population infected in some zones; famine, they explained, aggravated the situation. Returning to Freetown a few weeks later, they got to work with the help of a thick stack of documents (more than 150 typed pages) sent over by Gaston Muraz, Eugène Jamot's successor as the director of the Service général autonome de la maladie du sommeil (General Autonomous Service for Sleeping Sickness Control; SGAMS) for AOF.[31] In their report, they recommended setting up a system modeled on the French service in the area of epidemic focus in eastern Sierra Leone.[32] Lourie, however, was already one step ahead: "very anxious to test [diamidines] personally,"[33] he offered to launch the preliminary phase of the program—a trial of May & Baker's new compound—at once. If it "prove[d] to be of value," Lourie hoped, the drug might "considerably simplify the problem of dealing with the present, and other, outbreaks of sleeping sickness."[34]

The sleeping sickness campaign launched in Sierra Leone instantiated an *experimental* form of public health. These were the defining features of this experiment: a dramatic epidemic provided the pretext for a clinical trial, which in turn made available resources for treating the sick, described as "people of a particularly poor and undernourished type."[35] The medical campaign was entrusted to a researcher sent from the metropole, whose salary was paid by the

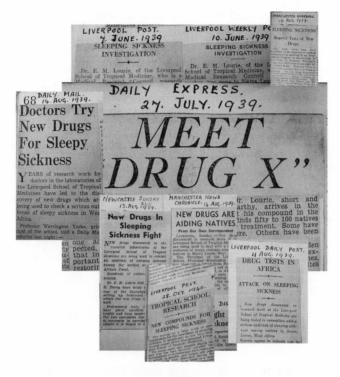

MRC and who had no experience with "colonial culture" or collective medicine. The campaign relied on a medical infrastructure created from scratch, directly imported from a neighboring colony, and tested for this purpose. The entire episode was broadcast to the public from the outset. Warrington Yorke, who was just about to leave for a conference tour in the United States, convened the British press in August 1939. "I cannot divulge the nature of the discovery," he announced, but there was hope: "new drugs discovered in the research laboratories of the Liverpool School of Tropical Medicine are to be used to conquer an epidemic of sleeping sickness among natives of the [w]est coast of Africa. Two Liverpool specialists . . . are setting up treatment centres. Tests have given excellent immediate results."[36] Fifteen or so English dailies, including the *Daily Express*, relayed the news.

Planned to last only a few months, Lourie's stay in Sierra Leone was extended to two years, the amount of time needed to prove the efficacy of diamidines and to fall out with the whole colony: it was said of him, using the French term, that he was *difficile* (difficult).[37] The first good news from the trial arrived in the fall of 1939, just as war broke out. Over the next few months, between worried letters about the threat of U-boats to maritime traffic and the bombing of Liverpool, Yorke kept an eye on the experiments. He pressed May & Baker to obtain additional samples, proposed new leads—trying diamidines to treat yaws, for example—negotiated for MRC support with Dale, and did his best to ease tensions between Lourie and the local medical service, even calling, when needed, on his connections at the Colonial Office.[38] Lourie's "pig-headed obstinacy" created complications in the control program he was meant to oversee.[39] He set up complex comparisons between treatment protocols, jealously guarded his files, and insisted on the long-term follow-up of patients to monitor for relapses—fine-grained details that were incompatible with the rhythms of a mass campaign *à la française*.

Miracle as Evidence

Across the empire, positive clinical results accumulated and made their way back to Warrington Yorke with words of gratitude for having "kindly provided" samples of diamidines.[40] In early 1940, Yorke announced the good news to the Royal Society of Tropical Medicine and Hygiene in London.[41] He had just received, he explained, a letter on the trial conducted in the hinterland of Sierra Leone. Lourie had written: "Trypanosomes and symptoms disappeared remarkably quickly in cases treated by the new compounds, and the speed with which many very late and almost moribund cases have recovered has obviously made an enormous impression on the local populace."[42] A letter Yorke received a few days later from Sudan, where Dr. Robert Kirk had tested stilbamidine in kala azar, was equally optimistic: "Three [patients I provisionally cured] have been clamouring for discharge for the last month, and have in fact been using the hospital only as a sleeping place from which they issue daily on a round of revelry—drinking, whoring, and generally beating the place up. While I personally pay more attention to weight records, blood counts and spleen punctures, the fact that these patients are able to behave in this fashion is regarded locally as convincing evidence that they have been very effectively restored to health and strength."[43] Yorke, though he was "very anxious to avoid extravagant claims," was congratulated. British chemotherapy was now in possession of new wonder drugs.

The adverse effects reported in some of the first patients put under treatment were appreciable, however; they included dizziness, fainting, and generally feeling unwell. When pentamidine was injected intravenously, patients complained of a sudden sensation of heat in the whole body, followed by itching and uncontrollable scratching, "particularly in the genital area," noted a doctor based in Uganda.[44] Some began to sweat or salivate profusely; others vomited or were incontinent. Yet comparisons with existing treatments decided in the diamidines' favor. Intramuscular injection seemed to attenuate the adverse effects, particularly with pentamidine, making it possible to complete a course of treatment for patients in the early stage of sleeping sickness in only a few days, as opposed to several weeks with previous therapies. Even when the first case of sudden death in the course of pentamidine treatment was reported in 1944,[45] the consensus was not revised: pentamidine by intramuscular injection was the new treatment of choice.

Under these circumstances, the results obtained by Emanuel Lourie, who returned to Britain in 1942, went almost unnoticed. His data were impressive in both quantity (more than three thousand patients monitored over two years) and quality: the sophistication of his statistical analyses was unrivaled in the field.[46] Yet his conclusions merely confirmed the superiority of diamidine compounds, which was hardly surprising or significant after so many positive results had already been published in 1939 and 1940.[47]

The compounds gained definitive trust in 1943, when a "European"—a Polish soldier being treated in a British hospital—was cured of trypanosomiasis, which he had caught in Sierra Leone, by pentamidine injections.[48] Although thousands of African patients had already given proof of similar results, this "premiere" justified a special publication in the British Medical Journal, thus making explicit the hierarchies that ordered imperial experiments: mice, rabbits, paralyzed syphilitics, Hindu seamen, African natives, and Whites.

On April 24, 1943, Warrington Yorke, the patron and source of inspiration for this series of experiments, died suddenly in his house in Birkenhead, a wealthy suburb of Liverpool. A Department of Chemotherapy was immediately created in his memory at the Liverpool School, thus sanctioning a long-standing emphasis on tropical pharmaceutical research. Emanuel Lourie, whose career was launched by the experimentation with diamidine compounds, was given the post of director.[49] The time for writing history had come: in a conference paper published in the British Medical Journal, Sir Henry Dale placed the discovery of diamidines between Ehrlich and sulfa drugs as one of the great moments in the history of modern therapeutic science.[50]

A very common feature with pentamidine . . . has been itching. This appeared precipitately immediately after injection, lasting for some minutes; it was generalized and often very pronounced, the grotesque antics of the patient, trying to scratch every part of his body simultaneously, being a source of great amusement to his companions.

E. M. Lourie, "Treatment of Sleeping Sickness in Sierra Leone," *Annals of Tropical Medicine and Parasitology* 36 (1942), 113–31, 119.

Experiments without Borders

Pentamidine experimentation was a transnational affair. It depended on exchanges between medical experts that crossed imperial lines. Inspired by the experiment of a Hungarian pharmacologist, discovered by British chemotherapy, tested as a chemoprophylactic by Belgian colonial doctors, and enthusiastically adopted by French and Portuguese mobile medical teams, pentamidine stimulated unprecedented competition and interaction. To reconstruct its biography, I have had to break out of the "protonationalist" frame adopted by many historical studies of colonial medicine, which confine their scope to a single colony or empire.[1] As a world war unfolded, colonial Africa became an experimental space that blurred the borders between empires, states, and pharmaceutical firms. The most important episodes in the experimental history of pentamidine, those in which its prophylactic effects (not just its curative properties, as before) were demonstrated, must be described and analyzed beyond the limits of the British Empire, along pathways of scientific exchange that mixed commercial interests, small talk, and chauvinism.

The Belgian Invention of Preventive Pentamidine

"As we have, in Léopoldville, exceptional conditions for the trial of products relevant to parasitology, I will always welcome with pleasure those you wish to entrust to me," wrote General-Doctor Lucien Van Hoof,[2] the head of the Belgian Congo's health service, on June 30, 1943, to Arthur Ewins, a May & Baker chemist, thanking him for his "shipment of 150 grams of pentamidine."[3] The war had redrawn the global map of tropical medical research: cut off from Brussels, doctors from the Belgian Congo were integrated de facto into the Allied camp. London, the headquarters for Belgium's government-in-exile, functioned as its metropole. These were the circumstances of the discovery of pentamidine's preventive effects in Léopoldville.

Posted in Congo since the end of the First World War, Van Hoof was among the world's top trypanosomiasis experts and one of the few scientists who mastered every phase of intervention into the disease, from animal testing to mass treatment campaigns. Along with a small circle of other experts, he was a familiar figure at international conferences on the subject.[4] Despite his military and administrative duties (he was appointed head of the colony's health service in 1934), he continued to pursue a research program in the spacious laboratories of the Institut de médecine tropicale Princesse Astrid (Princess Astrid Institute of Tropical Medicine) in Léopoldville, a flagship institution of Belgian colonial science established in 1937. There was no comparable site in Africa for trypanosomiasis research, partly because of Belgian doctors' expertise and international connections, but also thanks to the nearby availability of patients in a vast segregation camp located above the city.[5]

When Van Hoof received his first drug samples from May & Baker in early 1941, the therapeutic value of pentamidine was already well established. In May 1941, Van Hoof set about to evaluate its *preventive* effects. He worked with Dr. C. Henrard, a doctor at the institute, and Ms. E. Peel, a nurse lab technician. After conducting conclusive trials in guinea pigs, they set up a simple experiment: two "native volunteers" who had never been infected with sleeping sickness received an injection of pentamidine. Then, "every two or three days" for more than a year, the men were exposed to the bites of laboratory-reared tsetse flies. Week after week, "Moya and Bonkumu"—the reports referred to the subjects only by their first names—submitted to blood tests and lumbar punctures to test for infection. The men became familiar with the lab; offering up their bodies for experimentation was, for Moya and Bonkumu, a daily job. In June 1942, ten months after the prophylactic injection, trypanosomes were detected in Moya's blood. Two months later, Bonkumu was also diagnosed as positive. Van Hoof and his assistants thus concluded that pentamidine protection lasts nearly a year; only then did they treat their subjects with Bayer 205.[6] This success encouraged Van Hoof, who proposed even more "daring" experiments to May & Baker. Why not test, he suggested, the protective effects of pentamidine against malaria by subjecting some "natives" to injections of infected blood?[7]

To publish these results, Lucien Van Hoof called on an acquaintance, Dr. Clement Chesterman, who had previously worked as a Baptist missionary in the Belgian Congo and was now based in London at the Royal Society of Tropical Medicine. Chesterman had played a major role in Congo's medical history, notably by participating, from his Yakusu hospital near Stanleyville, in trypanosomiasis drug tests and treatment campaigns in the 1920s.[8] After returning to England in 1936, he continued throughout the war to mediate between anglophone and francophone, British and Belgian missionary and scientific worlds. He had put Van Hoof in contact with May & Baker; now he arranged for the publication of Van Hoof's article in the *Transactions of the Royal Society of Tropical Medicine*.

Published in February 1944, Van Hoof's findings were immediately criticized, especially by experts in Liverpool. Because he had failed to include control subjects, and thus to prove with certainty that the tsetse flies of the Léopoldville laboratory remained infective for the duration of the experiment, it was impossible to draw a conclusion about the protective power of pentamidine.[9] Furthermore, because the subjects were exposed to glossina bites immediately, that is, the day after the injection, it was possible that they had developed immunity to the trypanosomes early on, when the concentration of pentamidine in their blood was still high. These weaknesses in the design of the experiment were blatant, especially given that the unpredictability of experimental infection models was a known obstacle to designing reliable chemoprophylaxis trials.[10] Even after another, more elaborate study was conducted in 1945 with three new Congolese volunteers, it was still not demonstrated conclusively that pentamidine conferred *individual* protection.[11]

Doubts were supposed to be lifted by the "massive trials" launched in rural areas beginning in December 1942. These took advantage of the particularly well-oiled medico-administrative machinery of the Belgian Congo's sleeping sickness control services. A large-scale trial was set up in two villages of the Kwango district, about 600 kilometers from the capital in the heart of an epidemic focus zone that doctors crisscrossed on a regular basis. The local sleeping sickness control team was provided with a flask of 100 grams of pentamidine. Having first screened all inhabitants of the selected villages and "excluded from the trial" about a hundred positively diagnosed individuals, they selected about a thousand "healthy natives." These were divided into two groups; two-thirds of the subjects were given an intramuscular injection of pentamidine, while the remaining one-third served as a control group.[12] Six months later, no new case had been diagnosed in the injected group, while several control subjects were found to be infected. The trial was deemed a success, which was confirmed when the team, supplied with pentamidine from England, did its next rounds. "It seems to be shown by this experiment (the first executed in a rural area) that Pentamidine protects for 6 months but should be injected, out of precaution, every 3 months,"[13] concluded the supervisor of the trial in his report. In 1946 Van Hoof, in the article he published on the basis of the same data, stated more definitely that a dose of pentamidine protects "for at least six months."[14]

"The Saying Goes That in the Congo a Tribe of Pygmies Has Done the Work of Giants"

Belgian colonial doctors *wanted* to believe in the preventive power of pentamidine. For more than two decades, they had already been pursuing chemoprophylactic control strategies. As early as 1925, they had tested the preventive treatment of a healthy population with intravenous injections of Bayer 205 (even before its efficacy had been demonstrated in animals).[15] In the 1930s, these trials were repeated in various regions of Congo with ambiguous results, which the French and British contested: the protective benefits did not seem to last very long, while injections were followed by unpleasant side effects. The treatment also appeared, in the long run, to create favorable conditions for the emergence of cases of sleeping sickness called "cryptic infections," which were particularly difficult to detect and to cure.[16] Yet "Bayerization," as the Belgians called the technique, had its virtues: it was a "shock treatment" that allowed for lighter, faster campaigns focused mainly on the task of injecting. Furthermore, by radically disrupting transmission at the population level, it held the promise of rapid eradication. Finally, in the face of French and British skepticism, Bayerization's success designated it as a truly Belgian method, modest yet ambitious. Thus, the preventive use of pentamidine was, from the outset, seen as a mere variant of the Belgians' chosen approach. They even spoke in the first trials of "experimental Bayerization with MB 800";[17] the neologism "pentamidinization" appeared only in 1945.

This backstory explains why May & Baker's new drug elicited such enthusiasm in Léopoldville. It fueled the hopes of those already invested in Bayerization by offering new practical advantages: pentamidine protected for at least twice as long, intramuscular injections were much easier and quicker to administer than intravenous ones, and in prophylactic doses the drug caused not the "least intolerance."[18] Last but not least, the English compound was much cheaper.[19] Given Belgian doctors' plans to "Bayeriz[e] entire regions,"[20] the choice was clear. From 1943, trials of preventive pentamidine proliferated across the Belgian Congo.

The history of pentamidine highlights the strategic role played by the Belgian Congo on the Allied side in medical and other fields—alongside its more familiar contributions to the Allied victory as a source of labor, rubber, and uranium. The "colony," which in fact was autonomous during the war, operated as a laboratory of modernity that turned toward the United States, Great Britain, and the South African Union. It was an experimental site whose ambiguous status gave entrepreneurs like Van Hoof a remarkable degree of freedom, as well as access to technical and economic resources not available in Europe at the time, especially not in occupied Belgium. This dynamism was enacted and revealed in the creation in January 1942 of the journal *Recueil de Travaux de Sciences Médicales au Congo Belge* (Collected works of medical sciences in the Belgian Congo), the aim of which was to "prevent scientific studies conducted in the Congo from losing their timeliness due to overly lengthy delays in publication."[21]

Traveling frequently to the United States, Belgian colonial doctors managed to adapt penicillin production techniques in Congo, taking this opportunity to rename it Astridine, "the Congolese variety of the miracle drug."[22] They tested sulfa drugs as early as 1941 and DDT provided by American military research; they also launched quinine production on an industrial scale in Kivu. The large-scale experimentation with pentamidine was part of this series of military-scientific initiatives. In January 1944, during a tour of British Africa, Van Hoof announced through local newspapers the "excellent results obtained in [sleeping sickness] by injections [of an] English product called pentamidine and used [in] large quantities in Belgian colonial troops and native populations."[23] In July 1944, he concluded an interview on Radio Congo Belge by promoting his own article. "Do not think," he said, "that the Congo will lag behind the progress of medical science. Despite all manner of difficulties, the Service d'hygiène [Public Health Service] has just published a new issue of its *Bulletin des Sciences Médicales* [*Bulletin of Medical Sciences*]. Here is another copy of an English journal, the *Transactions of the Royal Society of Tropical Medicine and Hygiene*, which contains an article about the spectacular results obtained in the Congo in preventing and treating sleeping sickness with pentamidine."[24]

Returning to Belgium after the war to take up a position as professor at the School of Tropical Medicine in Antwerp, Lucien Van Hoof was invited to give the prestigious Chadwick Lecture at the Royal Society of Tropical Medicine and Hygiene on February 20, 1947. The former colonial doctor, who had risen to the top of his discipline, summed up in English his experience in the Belgian Congo: "the general use of preventive drugs, Bayer 205, and more especially the diamidines, is the most effective method we possess at present for fighting the endemic trypanosomiasis. . . . We have had proof that this method, when applied by adequate personnel with the necessary care, can bring about a complete eradication of the circulating parasite in man within 18 months, in a limited area."[25] Clement Chesterman spoke from the audience, greeting his "old friend" and praising the colonial achievements of the small Belgian nation, "a tribe of Pygmies [that] has done the work of giants."[26] Liverpool scientists, led by Lourie, were also present; they expressed skepticism about the method's principle, yet recognized the successful outcome of the mass trials.

The experiments with preventive pentamidine could now be launched on the scale of entire regions. Bayer 205 was gradually abandoned, and kilograms of pentamidine made their way to the stocks of the Belgian Congo's health services.

Pentamidine, Cinzano, and the Social Life of Doctors

Léopoldville, October 19, 1945

General Van Hoof arrived . . . very pleasant & speaks good English. He took me off to his office, we talked [sleeping sickness] for an hour. Then . . . Mount Leopold where Stanley [drew] his map & where we got a fine view of the rapids. Onto a [sleeping sickness] hospital & saw cases & the results of treatment. Wrote it up. At 11:40 left the hospital and made for the lab & met Drs. Henrard, Neujean, Mlle Peel. Chatted to them for a short time and then Van Hoof drove me back to the hotel. Had lunch with a Sabena pilot . . . walk[ed] around town for an hour. Lots of American goods in shops. . . . met a Canadian businessman with whom I had a very interesting chat. He thinks Belgian Congo is going to be one of the richest countries in the world because 90% of the world's uranium is there, endless amounts of industrial diamonds & about the finest waterway in the world.[27]

Pentamidine experimentation was based on a network of exchange made up of direct contacts between the "bush doctors," who traded the new powder among themselves. Drug tests were thus enmeshed in specific instances of colonial sociability: stories of men and sundowners, featuring the foot soldiers and big names of French, Belgian, and British colonial medicine.

Gaston Muraz witnessed the first British attempts to use diamidines when he met up with his colleague Emanuel Lourie at the Guinean border in 1939;[28] indeed, Muraz gave advice to the Liverpool scientists about infrastructure for the large-scale trial in Sierra Leone. The first French therapeutic trials followed from contacts with British colonial doctors.[29] In Bobo-Dioulasso, French experimenters used pentamidine and propamidine that had been offered as a "gift" by Nigeria's sleeping sickness service.[30] And so a few grams made their way across the interface of the British and French Empires, bringing along a constellation of knowledge, practices, and lifestyles.

Thomas Davey, who directed Alfred Jones's laboratory in Sierra Leone and set up the first trials of diamidines with Lourie, returned ill and exhausted to Liverpool in 1943. By the end of the war, he had recovered and been promoted to professor at the Liverpool School's main campus. In 1945, he set off on a long study trip in the African colonies at the request of the Colonial Office. One of his stops was in Bobo-Dioulasso, the site of the "control center" for sleeping sickness services across French Africa. He was welcomed by Dr. L. Nodenot, a colonial military doctor who had just tried pentamidine there. They spoke for many hours—so many that Davey later complained he "could not sleep for an hour; . . . was translating into French all this time."[31] His itinerary led to Abidjan, Bamako, Dakar, and Léopoldville, where he was received by Van Hoof; he then crossed the river to Brazzaville and chatted for two long hours about sleeping sickness in AEF with Dr. Jean Ceccaldi, the head of the control services for the colonial federation. At each stop, he carefully wrote down his impressions of each colonial service's methods and results, and also recorded the quality of the bed bases and mosquito netting; he described, by way of menus, the champagne, mushroom omelets, and Cinzano he shared with French and Belgian doctors and administrators. The history of colonial public health is made up of these forms of sociability, as described, for example, in the literary work of Dr. Destouches, alias Céline.[32]

Expertise on medicines traveled through such instances of mingling and exchange. The Belgians' success inspired the British who, from 1944, launched mass prophylactic trials of May & Baker's pentamidine in Nigeria, while the French across the Congo River in Brazzaville soon entrusted a young doctor with the task of running a trial in Nola, Oubangui-Chari (in AEF).[33] As therapeutic knowledge was transmitted, an international fraternity was brought into being; it was founded on a shared life "in the bush" and on conversations about the future of Africa and the backwardness of the "natives."

The Pharmaceutical Industry's Transnational Geographies

Pentamidine's tale is conducive to patriotic histories: the molecule was British, its method of administration was Belgian, and, to the great relief of French colonial doctors, the drug was about to become French. Yet the world of the pharmaceutical industry had its own geography, which unsettled national reference points. The relationships created through pentamidine testing during the Second World War drew the contours of a unique scientific network, connecting a Belgian colonial doctor, a former English missionary, and a London-based pharmaceutical firm, whose medical advisor, Dr. Robert Forgan, happened to be a former leader of the British fascist party.

More important, May & Baker, a flagship of British industry, had become a branch of the very French firm Rhône-Poulenc in 1927. The relationship between the companies was instigated so that they could join forces in competing against the German industry; the merger was designed to open up the captive markets of empire for products bearing both their brands.[34] This was a subtle arrangement, in which French control of the British firm was kept under the radar, secret even, so that May & Baker could retain the full benefit of its "national" status as it sold products from Rhône-Poulenc in the British Empire. Other than that, it was mostly a matter of company heads serving in each other's administrative councils and, of course, sharing their technical processes and patents. The Dagenham factory, built in 1934 and modeled directly on the factory in Saint-Fons, was one product of this Franco-British collaboration.[35]

The firms were joined by a tight mesh of scientific connections that wove through the Institut Pasteur and its colonial branches, the laboratories and factories of Rhône-Poulenc in the Paris region, those of May & Baker in Dagenham, and finally the Liverpool School and its colonial outposts in Sierra Leone and the Gambia. Diamidines animated this network, which beginning in the interwar period attracted major scientific figures, such as Ernest Fourneau.

In February 1939, Ewins began sending diamidine compounds to his correspondents at Spécia, the pharmaceutical division of Rhône-Poulenc, which in turn shipped them out to the French colonies.[36] With the war forcing May & Baker to operate more autonomously, the connection between the firms loosened. Pressed, under the occupation, by the German firm I. G. Farben to reveal information about Rhône-Poulenc's latest innovations, the French remained silent about diamidine compounds under the reasoning that they were "English" products.[37] Spécia then apparently managed, by following Ewins's instructions, to synthesize a small quantity of MB 800, which it renamed 2512 RP. In late 1942, Colonel-Doctor Jules Le Rouzic, the director of the sleeping control services for AOF, headquartered in Bobo-Dioulasso, placed an order for three thousand ampules. Just then, contact was broken between Vichy France and the colonies, and he never received the drugs. By the fall of 1945, the situation was back to normal, and the factory at Vitry-sur-Seine began producing one kilogram of pentamidine every week for "African experimenters," that is, for doctors in the French colonies.[38] In late 1946, AOF followed AEF and the Belgian Congo in launching its first trials of chemoprophylaxis; these affected nearly two thousand individuals in five villages in Guinea and two in Casamance. Business and science were flourishing.

Lomidine, a French Story

Meanwhile in Paris, French physicians were deciding that one of their own was the real inventor, or so it was said, of preventive pentamidine: Léon Launoy, a professor at the Faculté de pharmacie de Paris (Faculty of Pharmacy of Paris) and the scientific director of Spécia.[39]

Launoy had received samples of May & Baker diamidines from Ewins just before the war broke out in France.[40] Launoy was at that time obsessed with the question of preventive drug effects and immediately tested Ewins's compounds in vivo to assess their protective power. The results were somewhat promising: rats injected with high doses of pentamidine were resistant to trypanosome infection for several weeks. The results, published in the *Bulletin de la Société de Pathologie Exotique* (*Bulletin of the Society of Tropical Pathology*) in 1940,[41] almost certainly never made their way to Liverpool or Léopoldville, where Van Hoof was launching the experiments that would give him credit as the pioneer of preventive pentamidine.

Left out of the first retrospective accounts of the discovery, Launoy (who worked with a woman, Ms. Marie Prieur, but she rarely makes it into historical accounts) had to engage in the unpleasant task of staking a "claim to anteriority," which he slipped in as a footnote to a 1946 article. "We were surprised to note," he writes, "that J.-D. Fulton does not mention our study published on May 8, 1940, in the *Bulletin de la Société de Pathologie Exotique*. The circumstances of the last few years no doubt did not allow . . . [him] to become aware of our publication. . . . It is no less true that the first study pertaining to the preventive properties of aromatic diamidines . . . was published by us, five years ago. We believe that the priority of the demonstration of the prophylactic action of [the] above-mentioned diamidines is to be credited to us."[42]

At the time, Léon Launoy occupied a pivotal position in French pharmaceutical research: at the intersection of the colonial world, the pharmaceutical industry, and metropolitan scientific networks. A pharmacist by training, as

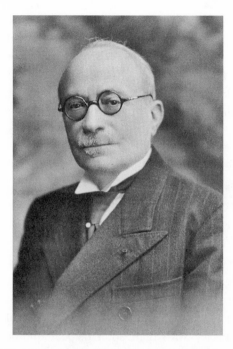

Léon Launoy (1876–1971). © Bibliothèque de l'Académie nationale de médecine.

well as an accomplished naturalist, he held multiple positions and honors: as the chair in zoology at the Faculté de pharmacie de Paris since 1938, he was also the scientific director at Spécia, which had hired him in 1927 after a stint at the Institut Pasteur. In his Spécia laboratory, Launoy systematized in vivo drug testing based on quantitative tests of toxicity and efficacy in small animals (rats, mice, rabbits); he was among the first to give experimental biology a central role in medical research and industrial production.

Launoy was also, like Warrington Yorke in Liverpool, an imperial scientist. Although he had never set foot in the colonies, Launoy maintained close connections with doctors in Africa, both for his work at Spécia and for his personal research program. He approached the trypanosome, as Yorke and Ewins had, as both a research topic and a laboratory testing device; being easy to cultivate and to observe, the parasite was useful in initial screening tests for biological activity in chemotherapeutic agents. Launoy was a passionate admirer of Jamot's initiatives (the latter's propaganda films were paid for by Spécia, and Jamot's teams went through kilos of atoxyl, stovarsol, and tryparsamide). Launoy directly ordered field doctors in AEF to conduct clinical trials and gave himself the role of commentator and propagandist for the French colonial enterprise.[43] He spoke at the Paris Colonial Exhibition of 1931 and welcomed content on Africa in the journal he edited, *Biologie Médicale* (*Medical Biology*); he was also a regular contributor to the *Annales Coloniales Quotidiennes* (*Daily Annals of the Colonies*). Sleeping sickness control was his favorite topic for popularization. "In Cameroon, Togo and AEF, the colonial enterprise of our humane France should not have as its shroud the undulating membrane of a trypanosome," he wrote in 1929;[44] the new means provided by the chemical industry heralded a "time when new infections will be reduced to a tiny number."[45] "In the colonies, the natives of all races must be confronted with the scientific truth"; scientists were to take on the mission of translating this truth into "brief and adequate orders," he explained in an article entitled "Instruire l'autochtone" ("Instructing the Native").[46] Launoy, who was awarded the Legion of Honor by the minister of colonies himself in 1928, was thus in a strategic position, one that connected Parisian science to the colonial field—or rather, one that revealed the impossibility of conceiving of these as separate universes. In the twentieth century, medical research was fundamentally a science of empire.[47]

Launoy was also the first historian of pentamidine: he gave himself the role of neglected precursor and retold his story of discovery in several articles. The contest over priority had no commercial or financial stakes. Rather, the goal was to insert the discovery of sleeping sickness chemoprophylaxis into the "great history of science" by producing an edifying account whose narrative arc would be neater than a succession of African experiments. By designating himself as the inventor of preventive pentamidine, Launoy relocated the new drug into his own universe. It was the discovery of a mandarin, an anointed expert, and one of the major figures of French biology and medicine.[48] It was the discovery of a scientist who was also a skilled writer, who had a passion for philosophical meditations on pure and applied science, and who cited Pasteur's aphorisms and passages from Claude Bernard's *Introduction à l'étude de la médecine expérimentale* (Introduction to the study of experimental medicine).[49] Launoy's historiographical efforts conferred the authority of "science" on a colonial technical innovation.

Launoy's writings placed pentamidine within a theoretical research program on chemical prophylaxis that had emerged in the late 1920s.[50] He gave the term a rigorous definition: chemical prophylaxis was not merely "anticipatory treatment,"[51] as in the case of taking daily doses of quinine, which

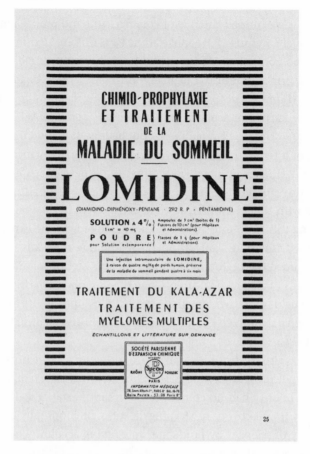

Publicity insert for Lomidine. *L'Essor Médical dans l'Union Française,* January 3, 1954, 25.

could be said to keep the drug present in the organism, awaiting the parasite. No, Launoy continued enthusiastically, chemoprophylaxis was nothing like "such day-to-day prevention,"[52] but was instead closer to a form of immunization, like vaccine therapy, which conferred durable protection with only "very small quantities" of a product.[53] Launoy opened up "chemical prevention" as a new frontier for the drug industry. At the same time, he gave unexpected legitimacy to colonial research by placing it at the forefront of this program. Animal experimentation would in fact come *after* trials in African people, inverting the usual order of research and implementation. "Being in contact with colonial doctors who lead the fight in the African bush and savanna, and who communicate to him the results obtained, Mr. Launoy can give his laboratory work a solid basis,"[54] the Pasteurian Constant Mathis aptly put it in 1949 before the Académie nationale de médecine (National Academy of Medicine).

Thus returned to its "rightful" place, the story of preventive pentamidine provided retrospective proof of the significance of Launoy's program and signaled medicine's entry into the era of chemical prevention. It gave Launoy a cascade of publications and honors in the postwar years. In 1949, his entire corpus was reprinted;[55] that same year, he was elected a member of the Académie nationale de médecine, and beginning in 1950, he presided over the Société de pathologie exotique (Society for Tropical Pathology). Now in the company of Claude Bernard, famous for intuitions and hypotheses, pentamidine was no longer just a colonial medicine; it was a French scientific achievement.

On December 4, 1946, the minister of health granted marketing authorization for 2512 RP, packaged in ampules of two cubic centimeters of solution and commercialized as "Lomidine."[56] The new drug, a methanesulfonate salt, was only a variant of the English pentamidine. Yet its launch, supervised by Launoy himself, was a kind of reward: the brand name Lomidine was likely chosen in homage to its inventor (Lo- for Launoy); it was a bit unsubtle perhaps, but Spécia specialized in such blunt wordplay in its selection of brand names.[57]

Lomidine was soon mass-produced: the factories of Vitry planned to synthesize 50 kilograms in 1947 just for the French colonies.[58] Across the French Empire, the paternity of the drug was no longer in question: "Professor Launoy can thus, without doubt, be considered the 'father' of diamidinization—I prefer the more euphonic term of Lomidinization—this method that has given and gives such wonderful results in French Black Africa," the colonial doctor Gaston Muraz asserted emphatically a few years later to the Académie nationale de médecine.[59]

CHAPTER THREE

The New Deal of Colonial Medicine

A new world was created in postwar Africa through the mobilization of a set of recent material objects, pentamidine among them. In just a few years, from 1945 to 1948, the new molecule had won over health authorities in the French, Belgian, Portuguese, and, to a lesser extent, British colonial administrations. The use of propamidine, one of the other drugs developed by May & Baker, was briefly envisaged by the Belgians but then abandoned following a trial that, while giving "marvelous" results,[1] caused numerous harmful incidents (miscarriages in particular). The neologism "propamidinization" was short-lived. Meanwhile, the Belgian trials of its sister molecule pentamidine had grown into life-size campaigns; by 1947, they affected more than a hundred thousand individuals.[2] Beginning in 1946, French and British trials confirmed the Belgian data: pentamidine seemed to have nothing but advantages. No new cases of sleeping sickness had been detected among the injected populations, the technique was simple, and no major accidents were reported. Of the family of diamidines discovered in Dagenham before the war, a single molecule remained. The hope of sleeping sickness control in Africa now depended on it.

Lomidinization (or pentamidinization), as preventive injections of pentamidine were now called, was defined as a priority strategy. Such enthusiasm cannot be explained merely as a self-evident and inevitable response to the substance's efficacy. The adoption of the drug also coincided with a turning point in colonial health policy, both revealing and accelerating a series of shifts. The first was a change in the scale of colonial states' intervention into African populations, which now made the conquest of tropical diseases a plausible goal. An unprecedented level of coordination among colonial powers provided the basis for a practical and institutional internationalization of colonial medicine. Finally, the use of coercion was stepped up to regain control over what doctors called the rising "indiscipline" of African populations. Pentamidine materialized but also contributed to the production of these broader trends. The new molecule rekindled a sense of ambition among doctors, elicited new forms of collaboration, and exacerbated the characteristic contradictions of late colonialism. In terms of the problems it created as much as those it resolved, the relationship between pentamidine and postwar colonial policies was, in the terminology of the sociology of science, one of coproduction.[3]

Pentamidine ushered colonial Africa into the era of international public health. It was also presented as a simple solution to the glaring contradictions of postwar colonialism. As colonial authorities' quest for modernization led to unanticipated and, in their view, worrying consequences—"political unrest" in particular—doctors also confronted growing protests from the populations they saw themselves as liberating from sickness and misery. How could the generous yet demanding enterprise of colonial public health be pursued at a time when coercion appeared to be simultaneously indispensable and illegitimate? As doctors' reactions wavered between resentment and outrage, pentamidinization offered a way out of the impasse. It promised to replace screening and long-term treatment, of which populations were growing weary, with an intensive push to prevent new infections. Pentamidine was a wonder drug for troubled times.

The Biopolitics of Development

In the postwar years, colonial health intervention faced a new order. This was to be an era of development and modernization, as announced in the British Empire by the Colonial Development and Welfare Act (1940) and in the French Empire by the Brazzaville Conference (1944). *Development* was the watchword: these empires sought to improve the living conditions of colonized populations and stimulate the economic growth of colonial territories. Thus conceptualized, development was to be concretized via massive transfers of funds from the metropoles, thus breaking away from the previously enforced principle of self-financing colonies, while experts—technocrats, scientists, doctors, and engineers—were to guide and plan political action. On the French side, this turn was reflected in the creation in 1946 of the Fonds d'investissement pour le développement économique et social (Economic and Social Investment Fund), financed in part by the Marshall Plan. This vision of development was coupled with a veritable material and technological revolution, marking this as an era of optimism: from the Jeep to DDT, from penicillin to the bulldozer, the Second World War was a test site for a series of technoscientific innovations, some of which were truly awe inspiring. Transposed from the military to the tropical world, these innovations opened up new possibilities for colonial states' interventions in populations and environments.[4]

Redefining colonialism in terms of development entailed reproblematizing the relationship among the health of populations, economic vitality, and the political future of colonialism, in other words, reworking what we might call, following Michel Foucault, colonial biopolitics.[5] Public health received unprecedented levels of support, which materialized in the creation of numerous institutions—a parade of acronyms and modernist buildings. It also extended its reach by mobilizing new forms of knowledge (demography and nutrition, for example) and techniques, opening up new fields of action (social welfare, for example) and recruiting a new generation of practitioners. As Fred Cooper and Vincent Bonnecase have shown,[6] there was a redefinition of the nature of the population itself as an object of study and intervention: the crude enumeration of census surveys and tax collection gave way to more sophisticated epidemiological, sociological, and economic knowledge of how African collectives worked. The transformation of indigenous populations' living conditions—which was to be evaluated with quantitative, universal standards of comparison—became the principal mission of colonial states.

A shared vision prevailed; it identified tropical diseases as the main obstacle to development and their eradication as the key to prosperity—and political stability.[7] In colonial settings, this line of reasoning was far from obvious: French colonial doctors, for example, had long and until recently been much more pessimistic about the relationship between economic growth and the improvement of public health. As late as 1945, one of the doctors at the head of Cameroon's health services wrote, echoing Jamot's earlier diatribes against the colonial economy: "We cannot at the same time exploit a country, develop it and remake its races."[8] With the same logic, some doctors called for the creation of states of humanitarian exception where the harsh laws of business and the economy might be suspended.[9]

The United States's extensive involvement in postwar international public health reformulated the nature of the problem: a coordinated war on tropical diseases thus came to be viewed as economic common sense.[10] Driven in part by Cold War concerns, the American approach was underpinned by a genuine economic and geopolitical doctrine, which would be reiterated by every president of this era, from Harry Truman's famous Point Four program to John F. Kennedy's creation of USAID (US Agency for International Development). According to this doctrine, technical solutions to the tropical disease problem could act as levers for transforming the tropical world, countering communist influence and securing the prosperity of the Western world. This approach posited an intimate connection between economic and medical progress; the first step toward development was to improve public health. "Health and productivity are indissociable concepts," wrote the French planners of the Ministry of Colonies in 1954, as if this was, by then, an obvious statement.[11]

The goal of eradication—the complete elimination of a disease or a vector—gave this program coherence and momentum.[12] The achievement of the total elimination of *Anopheles gambiae*, the mosquito vector of malaria, from Egypt and Brazil during the war conferred on eradicationism the status of a legitimate theory. By promising a return on investment, the target of eradication justified an intensive but rational effort, demanding a maximal extension of health-related action over space—for it was now necessary to reach entire populations. This radical stance also appealed to politicians and funders. Finally, eradicationism was propelled by a sense of technological messianism, with DDT, the synthetic insecticide tested on a large scale during the war, attaining resounding victories from 1944. This success inspired the malaria eradication program launched in 1952, which was paraded by the World Health Organization (WHO)—created just four years earlier—as its flagship program and which would continue to be an emblem of the eradication fever, the hopes, and then the disillusions of postwar international public health.[13]

The Reinvention of Mass Medicine

In the colonial world, doctors elaborated their own basic yet ambitious version of this conception of tropical disease through the spectacular implementation of a program of mass medicine. In the organizational model of sleeping sickness control, colonial mass medicine relegated economic and epidemiological subtleties to the background. "The idea is to organize a systematic offensive, we could say a 'Russian-style' offensive, . . . which is pursued until the enemy is eliminated, by attacking the causes of these great endemic diseases that obstruct the normal development of the black race and affect it both in numbers and in quality."[14] By defining its public health objectives in these terms during the Brazzaville Conference of 1944, the French government remained faithful to a population-based and racial model that had been well entrenched since the 1920s. Convened on the banks of the Congo River and attended by about fifty officials—for the most part, colonial administrators and members of the Algiers-based Comité de libération nationale (National Liberation Committee)

—the Brazzaville Conference is widely considered to be, for French Africa, the founding moment of "reformist colonialism." In the field of health, it ratified at the highest level the prioritization of mass medicine.[15]

The reasoning was clear, as laid out in the preamble of the plan adopted during the conference: "being accepted as a principle that the development of the race [is our] starting point, it seemed appropriate to put into effect a medical system able to protect and to treat not individuals but the masses."[16] The future was imagined in the (preexisting) form of a medicine of populations. Its methods would be collective, mobilizing mass campaigns and serial treatment, and its objectives would be demographic, aiming, as it was said in the interwar years, to "faire du noir,"[17] that is, to "multiply interventions in order to give to African races numerical value."[18] The target of medical action was the population itself: to prevent "social diseases" (at the time, the term encompassed tuberculosis, syphilis, malaria, leprosy, and sleeping sickness), the aim was to shrink, even to eliminate, the "virus reservoir" made up of carriers of a pathogen. The treatment of individuals was thus justified with reference to a preventive enterprise deployed on the collective scale. The vacillation that had long troubled colonial medicine—between a medicine of individual care and a medicine of mass prevention—seemed to have been resolved.

The main instigator of the conference's health proposals was Marcel Vaucel, a colonial doctor with many years' experience with sleeping sickness control in Africa.[19] Since 1940, Vaucel's star had been rising: as the head of Cameroon's Service de santé (Health Service), he joined the Free French Forces and accompanied General Leclerc's African campaign; in 1944, he was appointed the director of health services of the Commission for the Colonies in Algiers. He was not only a high-ranking Gaullist official, but also a respected authority on French tropical medicine. From Algiers, then a laboratory of French demographic and sanitary theory,[20] Vaucel identified sleeping sickness control as a model worth diffusing. The cornerstone of colonial public health, he proposed, would be a mobile, polyvalent, autonomous, and rigorously administered medical service modeled on sleeping sickness control teams.

The first decrees, published only a few weeks after the conference, created the Services généraux d'hygiène mobile et de prophylaxie (General Mobile Hygiene and Prophylaxis Services; SGHMP) in the federations of AOF and AEF and a Service d'hygiène mobile et de prophylaxie (Mobile Hygiene and Prophylaxis Service; SHMP) in Cameroon: thus began the era of *la médecine mobile* (mobile medicine), a term still remembered in Africa today.[21] Yet the new services were also written into a glorious history. The headquarters of the SGHMP for AOF, whose authority was meant to radiate across the whole federation, was located in Bobo-Dioulasso in Upper Volta in the buildings of the former sleeping sickness service created in 1939. Far from the federal capital of Dakar, this site inscribed the men of the SGHMP into the genealogy of great "bush doctors," such as Gaston Muraz. In a similar spirit, Brazzaville was chosen as the headquarters for the services for AEF, while in Cameroon, where the filiation with Jamot was direct, Vaucel predicted in his instructions to the governor that there already existed, in this historical home of mobile teams, "a method, an atmosphere and also materials that will make the head of [the] service's job easier."[22] The entire African territory of the Union française (French Union) was to be structured for mobile medicine and prophylaxis as a grid of sectors, drawing the contours of the sleeping sickness focus with little regard for administrative divisions. Each sector was to be supervised by a doctor and would have a logistical base, a place to stock medicines, park the mobile teams' trucks, and stack reports. As the colonies began receiving their first Jeeps, courtesy of the Marshall Plan, and as their road infrastructures improved rapidly, colonial medicine experienced a time-space compression. Entire regions were opened up to its reach; the era of medical tours on foot, with the doctor in a porter-carried chair, was about to end.

Mobile medicine was one of the priorities of the four-year plan for the equipping and modernization of the Territoires d'Outre-Mer (Overseas Territories); its section on public health was, from 1947, overseen by Marcel Vaucel. Appointed the director of the Service de santé at the Ministère de la France d'Outre-Mer (Ministry of Overseas France) after the liberation, and then, in 1952, the director of the Instituts Pasteur d'Outre-Mer (Overseas Pasteur Institutes),Vaucel was known as the boss of French colonial medicine throughout the 1950s. He orchestrated nominations and transfers, defined and negotiated agendas and budgets, all the while continuing to engage in cutting-edge scientific work. In his various roles, Vaucel took a leadership role in the conception and follow-up of Lomidinization campaigns. Viewed from his office, health policy and scientific expertise were indissociable: launching Lomidinization would help reinvent French colonial medicine. In 1944, weeks after the creation of the SGHMP, Vaucel dispatched from Algiers a circular on diamidines, along with translations of the Liverpool researchers' publications, to every health service in colonial Africa.[23]

Belgian colonial medicine took the same path. The reform of the Belgian

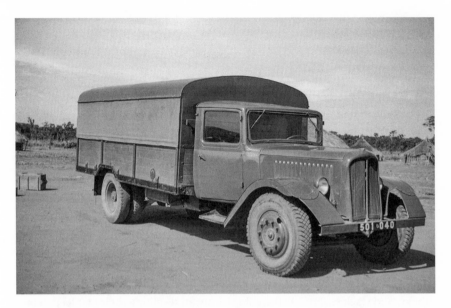

Truck used by an SGHMP Lomidinization team, Oubangui-Chari, 1956. Archives of
Marinette Lugagne.

Congo's health services, which took up an entire section of the ten-year economic and social development plan launched in 1949, was based on advice
from Albert Duren and Lucien Van Hoof, the Belgian inventor of preventive
pentamidine, who now held, since returning from Congo, the chair in tropical medicine at the Antwerp Institute of Tropical Medicine. The Van Hoof–
Duren plan, as it was then called, provided for massive investments in the
Belgian Congo's health and scientific infrastructure. The plan also, in its very
first paragraph, referred explicitly to the possibilities created by new "preventive
treatments" for sleeping sickness and malaria.[24] As in the French colonies, planners' blueprints materialized very quickly—such was the magic of the postwar
years. This was made possible by funding from the Fonds du bien-être indigène
(Fund for Native Welfare), created in 1947 with profits from the national lot-
tery. Pentamidinization campaigns in the Belgian Congo built on the practical
expertise of the FOREAMI (Fonds reine Elizabeth pour l'assistance médicale
aux indigènes; Queen Elizabeth Fund for Native Medical Services), a para-state
foundation to which the sanitary management of whole regions was delegated.
Integrated into a reorganized health service, the Belgian campaigns benefited
from the outset from unparalleled material and financial resources.[25]

In British Africa, trypanosomiasis specialists also played a major role in the design of public health and development policies; their ecological under-standing of the epidemic directly informed approaches to rural development in these regions.[26] Although the postwar British system relegated mobile med-icine to a secondary role, sleeping sickness control served, as in other colonies, as a resource for rethinking health action in the age of development.

These were utopian times. Fueled by experiments deployed across entire regions during the Second World War,[27] the ambitions of public health prac-titioners were immense and well publicized. Advertisements for Lomidine cir-culated on the glossy paper of imperial printing presses and official brochures.

An Epidemic of Indiscipline

The enthusiasm for preventive pentamidine was also a reaction to obstacles facing the new mass medicine. The sleeping sickness epidemic was flaring: the Allied armies' demand for rubber during the war had sparked a "rubber rush" across Africa's forested regions, especially after the Allied camp was cut off from the hevea latex supplied by the plantations of Java and Indochina. It had been known since the beginning of the twentieth century that gathering wild forest latex—the economic driver of the "red rubber" atrocities—created ideal conditions for epidemic outbreaks of trypanosomiasis.[28] The biggest wartime rubber exporters—the Belgian Congo, AEF, Cameroon, and Guinea—were the colonies with the strongest epidemic resurgence. Sleeping sickness had been brought under control by the late 1930s. Just a few years later, the threat of epidemics was reemerging from Angola to Casamance.

Sleeping sickness control services were, moreover, confronted with an epi-demic of indiscipline; the "growing license [taken by] populations,"[29] that is, an increasing tendency to avoid the colonizers' medical campaigns, jeopard-ized the entire program. Yet coercion no longer appeared to be a legitimate op-tion. Preventive pentamidine offered a way out of this impasse by promising to make screening and repeated treatment unnecessary in the near future. The new drug had, as Emanuel Lourie said pithily in 1944, "administrative advantages."[30]

At the time of the first trials in the Belgian Congo, Van Hoof had already made a link between the need to turn to chemoprophylaxis and the obsta-cles confronting older strategies: "the future of sleeping sickness control campaigns by sterilizing the human reservoir appears to be seriously compro-mised."[31] "After decades of encouraging results," the statistical curve was hit-ting a plateau. Emerging parasite resistance to arsenical drugs, such as atoxyl and tryparsamide, cast doubt on the very principle of mass campaigns, which aimed to work patiently, treating each trypanosome carrier, to pare down the virus reservoir. At the same time, the Belgian teams encountered another form of resistance: the opposition of "the natives." It was becoming harder and harder to count on a "disciplined population"; the British missionary Sir Clement Chesterman recalled nostalgically at the Royal Society "those days [when it was still] permissible to use the chicote, and [an uncooperative] Chief got the benefit of it."[32] This was a new era, and it needed a new technique. In the Belgian Congo, annual injections of pentamidine would allow the medical service, Van Hoof explained, to "economize time and labor" and to "limit the [the need for] convocations and comings and goings of the blacks."[33] As an era of disorder and development opened, preventive pentamidine appeared to be a miracle solution.

For postwar mass medicine, indiscipline was a critical issue. French doctors were very worried about "a profound change in the mentality of natives,"[34] which manifested in growing rates of absenteeism during campaigns. "Seeing [for themselves] that the dodgers are no longer being subjected to constraints or to sanctions, the natives dodge [the campaigns] in ever greater numbers," warned Raymond Beaudiment, the head of the SHMP in Cameroon, in 1946.[35]

The problem of indiscipline was addressed as a technical issue to be measured, mapped, and interpreted. The medico-administrative apparatus of mobile medicine was already focused on the "presence rate," the percentage of the population that showed up for visits from the mobile team. Seen as a measure of the popularity of colonial rule, the presence rate was especially the "target of the hygienist," that is, the precondition for successful widespread prophylaxis. Gaston Muraz thus remembered "sometimes order[ing] his] doctors to interrupt prospection [screening surveys] already underway if the index of presence at convocations did not reach 80%: [it was] a waste of time and money to leave behind unsterilized virus reservoirs."[36] When, in Eugène Jamot's time in Cameroon, the rates came close to hitting the 100 percent mark, "we were then absolutely sure of seeing just about the entire population, to let only a handful of infected individuals slip from our grasp, to shrink the virus reservoir to its minimum. . . . Today we consider ourselves lucky to get 80%, and sometimes [the rate] falls under 60%."[37]

Beginning in 1943, presence rates collapsed across French Africa. Doctors commented on this drop repeatedly in their reports, page after page, month after month. Attending to the details for each region and *groupement* (grouping),[38] they drew an ever finer-grained portrait of the menace; in other words, they ethnicized it. In Cameroon, "*terroirs* [hotbeds] of indiscipline," to paraphrase Achille Mbembe,[39] were designated. These overlapped with the political bases of the nationalist movement of the Union des populations du Cameroun (UPC; Union of the Peoples of Cameroon), such as Edéa, the Bamiléké area, and the city of Douala, which "beat every record" in 1950: "this is becoming ridiculous."[40] The prize went to the city's Bamiléké neighborhood, where the rate of presence fell as low as 25 percent: "this gives us an idea of how seriously this grouping takes the orders it is given."[41]

In AEF and AOF, the same type of cartography and ethnic logics were deployed. Colonies, circles, and cantons were scrutinized on the basis of numerical data. The situations in Senegal, Dahomey, and Togo were deemed acceptable with the exception of a few spots. In the northeast of the colony of Côte d'Ivoire, however, the SGHMP struggled in the face of the "legendary indiscipline of the Lobi."[42] In the regions of Danané and Man, the situation was explosive. The "population's overt ill will" prompted the dispatch of a special investigative mission by the administration and the interruption of a trial of preventive pentamidine underway in the area. The worst conditions were in Banfora; rates there dropped from "91% in 1944 . . . to 37% in 1947!"[43] Embedded in this analysis of indiscipline was a critique—a critique already prevalent among doctors working in British and Belgian Africa since the 1930s—of the uncontrollable consequences of colonial modernization.[44] The so-called floating population was at the heart of such anxieties. This category, drawn from nineteenth-century European demography, was applied in the African context to anyone who eluded ethnic and geographical assignment to a rural "tribe." The "floating population," which centered around cities and was fed by rural exodus, labor migration, and flight from forced labor during the war, inspired long passages in reports: it was uncontrollable, ungraspable, and, through a rebound effect, destabilized rural communities.

Back to Order

French doctors' condemnation of indiscipline was a cliché; now, however, they also proposed a political diagnosis, which was addressed to their superiors. Doctors explicitly protested a series of laws and decrees, enacted in the spring of 1946, that tore down some of the pillars of the old colonial system. For doctors, the Houphouët-Boigny Law, which abolished forced labor, and especially the law of May 7, 1946, known as the Lamine Gueye Law, which extended citizenship to the entire population of the empire and thereby, in principle, put an end to colonial subjection, weakened the foundation of medical authority. The abolition of the Code de l'indigénat (the regime of administrative sanctions applied to colonial subjects), which had included an obligation to submit to prophylaxis campaigns, revoked doctors' coercive powers. From Bobo-Dioulasso to rue Oudinot,[45] colonial doctors worried about the creation of a legal vacuum; they warned that liberalization of the colonial regime threatened the prophylactic enterprise as a whole.[46] As early as 1945, complaints were paired with demands for corrective steps. "These measures," Beaudiment explained, "may appear as a violation of personal liberties . . . but the stakes are too high to weigh the future of a territory against the respect of principles that are still beyond the grasp of insufficiently evolved populations."[47]

In 1946–47, colonial doctors' pleas made their way to the metropole via figures such as Gaston Muraz and Marcel Vaucel. The problem was debated by the Consultative Commission on Sleeping Sickness, which met at the Ministère des colonies in late 1947.[48] The commission identified the law of May 7, 1946, as a source of obstacles to the summoning of populations, and it recommended tougher sanctions on absenteeism, following the example set by AEF, which had adopted a new decree earlier in 1947.

In AOF, the problem was debated in some colonial assemblies, which rejected the option of reinstating the obligation to submit to medical screening.[49] In 1951, a justification of mass gatherings was found by declaring "imminent danger to public health"; this drew on an older exception, dating from the beginning of the century, which had been designed as a provision for major epidemics.[50] In Cameroon, the return to order was spectacular: two decrees, issued a year apart, instituted strict control over the mobility of the population and its presence during medical-screening operations. On June 13, 1947, the sanitary passport was reinstated for the residents of all zones known to be infected by trypanosomes (this applied to nearly the whole territory).[51] On June 1, 1948, a decree was published "making medical visits compulsory, with the aim of screening for endemic-epidemic diseases and the treatment of individuals known to be affected by these diseases." The legislative arsenal was now impressive, imposing the obligation to be screened, to be treated, and, for contagious individuals, to be "segregated"; infractions could be reported by doctors or by health assistants and could be "punished by imprisonment of 1 to 15 day[s], and a fine of 3,600 to 24,000 francs."[52] By 1948, members of the health services were optimistic: "disorder is on its way out."[53]

The legislative adoption of preventive pentamidine boosted doctors' morale. Of course, it would demand considerable organizational work; the problem of sleeping sickness was now "technically but not administratively resolved."[54] More important, the new technique seemed, almost beyond hope, to be capable of regaining control over some new factors of the sleeping sickness situation. These were the very aspects that doctors identified as disorders of modernization, such as transboundary worker migration and the concentration of the floating populations around cities. From the end of 1947, good news was announced. The first trials of pentamidine in Nigeria targeted mining camp workers, who frequently moved back and forth between villages and their workplaces.[55] Preventive injections succeeded in protecting and "sterilizing" this mobile population of potential disease carriers, with no need for protracted treatment and diligent follow-up—measures feasible only in sedentary populations. In AEF and the Belgian Congo, the new tactic was confirmed to be capable of treating transboundary epidemic focal areas where population control measures were unreliable.[56] In AOF, where the epidemic was concentrated in difficult-to-access forested regions, chemoprophylaxis kindled great hope; there were proposals to implement mass treatment along the main roads, where all travelers would be injected at "screening stations" akin to medical checkpoints.[57] The efficacy of pentamidine offered a simple solution to the problem of indiscipline: make Africans' consent irrelevant to their protection.

The adoption of pentamidine thus coincided with a return to order: on December 27, 1947, as the sleeping sickness commission's meeting on absenteeism drew to a close, Vaucel presented the results of chemoprophylaxis trials in AEF; they "exceeded all expectations."[58] At the same time that the excessive license of the "natives" had threatened the health of the empire, pentamidine promised to alleviate the symptoms of colonial disorder.

Inter-Imperial Blessings

The year 1948 opened with another Brazzaville Conference. From February 2 to 8, French, Belgian, British, South African, and Portuguese trypanosomiasis experts met in the capital of AEF for the first African Conference on Tsetse and Trypanosomiasis. Their objectives were to discuss the results attained in various colonies and to take stock of the latest advances.[59]

Commission number one, which was assigned the task of addressing medical issues, included most of the doctors who had supervised chemoprophylaxis trials in African colonies, including French colonial doctors, a British delegation led by Emanuel Lourie, and three Belgian colonial doctors. On its working agenda was the study of the "action of new trypanocides, of which some are likely . . . to profoundly alter the current modalities of sleeping sickness control, [or at] least to revitalize it."[60] The diamidines developed during the war in particular had attained "results [that] exceeded all expectations" in terms of both therapy and prophylaxis.[61] Reports of the trials in AEF, the Belgian Congo, and Nigeria had circulated in the months leading up to the conference. Approval was unanimous, and the commission recommended an expansion of "the application of chemical prophylaxis methods across the African territories in which sleeping sickness is endemic."[62] A standard posology was proposed. The adoption of pentamidine thus coincided with a pivotal moment in the internationalization of public health in Africa: this was the first time that a disease control strategy obtained consensus in an inter-imperial context. Pentamidinization was the first international mass medicine program in Africa.

Inter-imperial collaboration in tropical medicine was not a new phenomenon. It might even be said that doctors' exchanges across imperial borders were constitutive of the discipline from its birth. During the interwar years, the League of Nations had made sleeping sickness control a model of international collaboration.[63] Official correspondence intensified during the Second World War, when the Belgian and French colonies of Central Africa, cut off from their metropoles, joined the Allied camp and turned for their drug supplies to British colonies and to South Africa. The conference in Brazzaville also dovetailed with a series of meetings and conferences initiated in Lagos in 1943.[64]

The inter-imperial exchanges in Brazzaville, however, had a new performative function: at a time when colonial powers were coming under fire in the international arena, establishing collaborative medical endeavors served as a common defense of the "new colonialism" and its modernizing good faith. As Vincent Bonnecase has shown for other contemporary initiatives, this stance was also part of a strategy of playing off "colonial internationalism against international organizations."[65] Projects spearheaded by the World Health Organization, which was seeking to gain a foothold in Africa, were at that time a topic of worried correspondence between colonial authorities.

The new collaborative approach was implicitly contrasted with a past of nationalist bias. The Brazzaville recommendations, which were published in

1950 in a bilingual book, had an "objective quality," Vaucel explained when he returned to France, given that they "reflect[ed] the specific viewpoint of English, French and Belgian technicians who had worked for many years across all the sleeping sickness regions of black Africa."[66] In this respect, the introduction of pentamidine can also be seen as a declaration that the era of Germanin and Belganyl (the two national appellations, German and Belgian, respectively, of Bayer 205) was over. The time had come for friendly and technical exchanges. Taking advantage of his trip to the conference, James-Leslie McLetchie, the head of the sleeping sickness service of Nigeria, toured with the teams led by Commander-Doctor J. Chassain in the French Congo as they began their first preventive Lomidinization campaigns, and thus McLetchie learned the technique in the field.[67] Delegates to Brazzaville from the Portuguese colonies returned from the conference armed with new knowledge and ready to launch a large-scale pentamidinization campaign in Angola and Portuguese Guinea. Two Belgian doctors traveled to the Guinea border to train mobile teams from Angola.[68]

At the institutional level, the conference ratified the creation of an international organization devoted to sleeping sickness. The organization had a dual structure: the International Scientific Committee for Trypanosomiasis Research, whose role was to orient and coordinate research and whose secretariat was based in the Colonial Office in London, and the Permanent Inter-African Bureau for Tsetse and Trypanosomiasis (BPITT), which established its headquarters in Léopoldville in the offices of the Institut Princesse Astrid. The latter was to be jointly administered by the two Congos and codirected by the heads of the Institut Pasteur in Brazzaville and the Institut Princesse Astrid. Its mission was to facilitate the exchange of information on a continental scale by translating and disseminating scientific publications to a network of about a hundred correspondents. At this time, in February 1948, this extent of international coordination was unprecedented—neither malaria control, nor nutrition research, nor even smallpox vaccination programs had any comparable structure. These new institutions would serve as a model of collaboration in other fields.[69] The WHO, which would later put forward an alternative vision of international space, was not yet materially present. Thus for the first and, in some ways, for the last time, an inter-imperial form of scientific cooperation was instituted, with its headquarters in the heart of equatorial Africa.

Debates on pentamidine occupy a large portion of the archives generated by more than ten years' worth of BPITT activity; during the whole decade of the 1950s, the transmission of knowledge about the drug kept a documentary apparatus working full steam. The history of pentamidine thus is also a history of the typists and clerks of the Institut Princesse Astrid, which, by translating, copying, and recopying articles written by members of the network simultaneously communicated, legitimated, and stabilized trust in the new technique.

CHAPTER FOUR

The Spectacle of Eradication

A few years after the Second World War, the Ministère de la France d'Outre-Mer produced a document tallying up the achievements of sleeping sickness control in AOF:

53,087,283 individuals were examined

410,453 were found infected with trypanosomiasis

1,636,865 lumbar punctures were performed

8,134,005 injections of trypanocides were performed

9,977 kg of trypanocides were used

16,418,573 days of hospitalization were recorded

218,796 patients were cured

52,977 patients are on the path to recovery

819,016 individuals were subjected to chemoprophylaxis
    (Lomidinization)

122,247 hectares were decontaminated by agronomic prophylaxis

184,181 glossinas were dissected

Nestled in this list is what we might call the poetry of that era. This chapter reflects on an act repeated 819,016 times by 1952 in AOF and more than a million times across Africa before its colonies gained independence: the preventive injection in the buttocks of several cubic centimeters of Lomidine solution. The officials' enumeration did not just refer to enacted gestures, calculated to the nearest unit—the number of flies dissected or hectares cleared. It also participated in what Roland Barthes calls a higher-order language,[1] of which the signifier was that public health is part of a coherent and quantifiable enterprise; its goal, as well as its routine practice, is to produce numerical indicators that are comparable between imperial nations and can be mobilized to counter critiques of colonialism. The history, at once minute and gigantic, of the Lomidinization campaigns must thus be understood as both routine and a showcase of the new colonialism.

Making Numbers

Vast Lomidinization campaigns were launched across Africa following the intercolonial conference at Brazzaville in 1948. Then came accounts written in numbers: tables and graphs telling the story of cases of sleeping sickness becoming rarer; rates of prevalence and incidence dropping; the number of Lomidinized individuals soaring; and the percentages of "absents" and "non-compliants" subsiding.

Historians have learned to mistrust statistics. The figures produced by colonial states were technologies of government, tools for ordering populations; they were also monuments of empire and active producers of a "self-fulfilling" fiction "rather than principally referential to a complex reality external to the activities of the colonial state," as Arjun Appadurai has written.[2] My aim here is not to express irony or skepticism about the magnitude of the declared achievements—pentamidine injections were performed by the million, and there is no reason to doubt these figures. My aim, rather, is to grasp the performative dimension of the act of counting: what it meant, in the course of injection campaigns, to "make numbers" both in the sense that large-scale repetitions of a tricky medical gesture entailed organizational constraints and with reference to the burden imposed on the day-to-day work of mobile teams by the very acts of counting and accounting. In other words, I seek to understand the "feedback effects on the course of action" of numbers that did not merely document and measure this action,[3] and to understand how it mattered—for patients queuing up under the sun, for nurses filling up syringes, and for doctors typing up reports—to be part of an imperial statistic.

The numbers were impressive, "American-style" even, as one French doctor wrote in the publication *Marchés Coloniaux* (*Colonial Markets*).[4] The number of injections rose exponentially from 1946, when several thousand were recorded, to reach the two million mark for the year of 1953 alone. The sums were tallied on a regular basis in Bobo-Dioulasso and in Brazzaville at the headquarters of the SHMP and then transmitted up the chain of command to the BPITT in Léopoldville and to the Ministère de la France d'Outre-Mer in Paris, which archived the summary reports. After the mid-1950s, the numbers abated. By independence, twelve to thirteen million preventive pentamidine injections had been administered across Africa.[5]

These numbers also had a material existence: orders skyrocketed at the factory in Vitry-sur-Seine, which produced the powder for the French colonies, and in Dagenham, which supplied the Belgian Congo and the British colonies. The workers who prepared and packaged the drug (women, seen as neater and daintier, made up the majority of those entrusted with this task) had to step up their speed of production. From 1949, Spécia's orders exceeded 500 kilograms per year. Pushed to maximal capacity, production reached 70 kilograms per month, most of which was destined for the French colonies (which stockpiled hundreds of kilos) and the Belgian Congo. In 1952, doctors from the Portuguese colonies joined the list of clients; they inquired about the possibility of obtaining more than 100 kilograms—enough for five hundred thousand injections.[6]

Numbers also conceal an uneven spatial distribution of the campaigns, which were confined to fairly limited zones. The geography of Lomidinization followed the map of trypanosomiasis's endemic focal areas, but it was equally shaped by political logics and contingencies: by the competition between regions and colonies and between model territories and peripheral zones, as well as by the varying degrees of enthusiasm with which health services adopted the strategy, ranging from exaltation in the French and Portuguese colonies to skepticism in the British ones.

Lomidinized Africa

Cameroon was, without doubt, the African territory where Lomidinization was implemented with the greatest intensity. Formerly a German colony and then, from the interwar years, a League of Nations mandate, Cameroon was, beginning in 1945, a United Nations trust territory; its largest portion was placed under French administration, and a strip of land in the west, adjacent to Nigeria, was under British administration. As trustees of an "international colony," these administrations accounted for their "civilizing efforts" through carefully written and illustrated annual reports.[7] Eugène Jamot had, in his time, skillfully leveraged Cameroon's status—which increased the significance of public health action as a yardstick of the colonizers' benevolence—to obtain metropolitan financial support for his sleeping sickness control mission.[8] Caught in the rivalry between colonizing nations, Cameroon was, after 1945, treated as a showcase by France, which invested massively in its infrastructure and public health—comparatively much more, in terms of the ratio of funding to population, than in AEF or AOF.[9] Cameroon, both a laboratory of modernization and a land of historic sleeping sickness control, was overinvested by Lomidinization campaigns.

In the case of Cameroon, we can see how campaigns targeted both histori-cal focal areas of the disease and the new frontiers of the postwar epidemic in border zones and city outskirts, as well as groups of workers on plantations, at public works sites, and in mines. In November 1948, the first large-scale im-plementation of the strategy in Yokadouma in the eastern part of the territory was a resounding success: in a region ravaged by the epidemic, the preventive Lomidinization of its entire population caused the rates of incidence to plum-met from 14 percent to 0.8 percent. Whereas before the first round of injec-tions, more than four hundred new infected individuals had been recorded, only ten new cases were detected several months after, in early 1949.[10]

Over the space of three years, Lomidinization was extended to all disease focuses; the majority were well known, having been identified at the time of Jamot's mission, but additional areas that until recently had been free of the disease, such as the cities of Yaoundé and Douala, were also targeted. The treatment reached two hundred thousand individuals in 1952; the number of Lomidinized people unsurprisingly figured in the government's report to the United Nations, for which the entire propaganda apparatus had been mo-bilized. Lomidinization made it possible to regain control over an epidemic situation that had gotten out of hand in both the medical and political sense: on the territory's outer edges, the epidemic in Yokadouma was completely stamped out, while in Yaoundé, "with a population in which a spirit of com-pliance is not the dominant quality," reported the SHMP, "it seems that pre-ventive Lomidine offers us hope."[11]

The same logic was at work on the larger scales of the federations of AOF and AEF, where the number of injections exceeded a million in 1953 alone. The coverage of the campaigns mostly followed the existing grid of the SGHMP's "special sectors," which absorbed most of the resources. In AOF, preventive Lomidine was mainly used in the forested regions of Côte d'Ivoire, Guinea, and Casamance and much less in the older epidemic focuses of the savanna regions of Upper Volta, French Sudan, Dahomey, and Senegal.[12] In the latter regions, the epidemic, concentrated around gallery forests and water sources, had not flared up during the war, and the test-and-treat system, supported by an apparatus of patient records unparalleled in Africa—and a "naturally disci-plined population," doctors said[13]—worked well. Lomidinization opened the possibility of targeting mobile workers who traveled back and forth between Upper Volta and southern Côte d'Ivoire; perceived as threats to their home re-gions, these migrant workers were treated during regular visits to their sites of temporary residence in the south, in the so-called Mossi villages (that is, people from northern Côte d'Ivoire and Upper Volta).[14] Campaigns in AEF were essentially focused on epidemic focal areas known since the beginning of the century, which extended from the coast of Gabon to Chad, via Haute-Sangha in Oubangui-Chari, covering most of the French Congo. Mining and forestry companies ordered their own supplies of Lomidine from Spécia to protect their employees.[15] Lomidinization was adapted to the era of modern transportation: an aquatic motorized brigade was created to Lomidinize areas accessible only through waterways. Doctors reacted enthusiastically: "organization," they commented, "has replaced tourism and exploration."[16] Finally, along the corridor of the Congo River (the segment north of Brazzaville-Léopoldville), campaigns were coordinated with Belgian teams on the other bank to synchronize the treatment of an "unstable, indisciplined population constantly renewed by the influx of [individuals] fleeing either French or Belgian authority."[17] Beginning in 1949, teams injected Spécia's Lomidine on the right bank and May & Baker's Pentamidine on the left bank.

Pentamidinization was widely implemented by the health services of the Belgian Congo, which began organizing mass campaigns as early as 1946, ahead of other African territories. These campaigns covered Léopoldville province (extending across the whole southeast from the Lower Congo to Kwango), Katanga (where "foci [were] methodically decontaminated"),[18] Kasai, Kivu up to the valleys of the Ruzizi River (on the Ugandan border) and of the Uele River (on the border with the British Sudan), and Ruanda-Urundi.[19] The zone of Kwango, which was located near the site of the first trials of 1942 and which had been entrusted to the FOREAMI, served as both a showcase and a laboratory. This arid, underpopulated, and economically "useless" region had a high prevalence of sleeping sickness. Beginning in 1939, the FOREAMI selected Kwango as a pilot zone and concentrated its Congolese activities there, conducting regular medical surveys and demographic follow-up and establishing a dense network of maternity clinics and dispensaries. Kwango was among the few regions in Africa that came close to following the recommended six-month intervals for pentamidinization.[20]

In the British colonies, however, pentamidinization was applied more sparingly, for reasons I will come back to. Campaigns were confined to Sierra Leone, in the area where diamidines were tested during the war, and northern Nigeria, where tin mine workers were injected every six months.[21]

The most recent and most zealous converts were Portuguese doctors, who

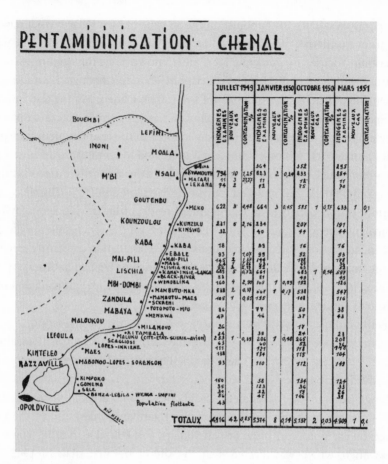

Franco-Belgian campaigns along the Congo River. "Rapport sur la situation sanitaire de la frontière franco-belge pendant l'année 1950" (4467/932). © Archives africaines, Brussels.

staked everything on "pentamidinização total." Following the conference in Brazzaville, they succeeded in persuading the government of Angola to launch a large-scale pentamidinization program.[22] In absolute figures, this would become Africa's most intensive operation; it was concentrated in the northwestern part of the territory, a diamond-mining area where the health services benefited from exceptionally high levels of resources.[23] In Portuguese Guinea, the health service also began to pentamidinize in 1949, just after the Brazzaville Conference; by the 1950s, it was using the method on a regular basis. In Mozambique, however, as in other East African sites, the trials failed: pentamidine did not appear to protect against *T. rhodesiense*, the parasite prevalent in East Africa.[24]

These campaigns were inseparable from a form of geographical imagination; the cartography of the epidemic and of the campaigns, with their ethnic-epidemiological entities (the focal areas), became the reality on which the health services acted. One report, for example, spoke of "two injections . . . [which] thus completely cleaned up the focus of Muzengo."[25] Villages, roads, cantons: these were the entities to be Lomidinized. Often it was noted, for the sake of brevity, in the column of a report corresponding to the name of a village or a region, quite simply "LT," which stood for *lomidinisation totale.*

Campaign Rhythms

For the chemoprophylactic team the man in charge, who is unlikely to be [a] doctor, must be a senior and highly responsible auxiliary. The principles of mass production and time and motion study should be invoked to ensure the maximum speed and efficiency in getting through, say, 250 injections in a morning. The man actually giving the injection should merely have to turn half around in order to hand over his used syringe and take a freshly charged one. Equally as he turns back again, a freshly iodined buttock, and the appropriate dose, should present themselves before him. Finally, the persons injected must be rubbed, led away to rest, and supervised. For all this, the team must consist of 1 dispenser, 1 injector, 1 man charging syringes, 1 man sterilizing syringes, 1 man preparing buttocks, 1 man doing aftercare on buttocks and setting patients at rest. All except the dispenser, the injector and the man responsible for surveillance of persons resting after injections can be intelligent labourers, even illiterates.[26]

Pentamidinization campaigns came close to achieving a form of standard medicine that, with its procedures rationalized in the extreme, was an archetype of what would later be called a "vertical public health program." An identical mode of operation was, with only minor variations, adopted across Africa. Pentamidinization began with the diagnostic screening of an entire population with clinical examinations and blood tests. Those found infected with trypanosomes were treated at once according to current therapeutic protocols, while all healthy subjects received a preventive dose of pentamidine injected into the buttock, followed by a few hours of compulsory rest. The process was, in theory, to be repeated every six months.

This protocol merely added a new module to the older organization of the sleeping sickness control campaigns conducted since the 1920s, in which the simplest gesture was codified.[27] The rationalization of work, often displayed

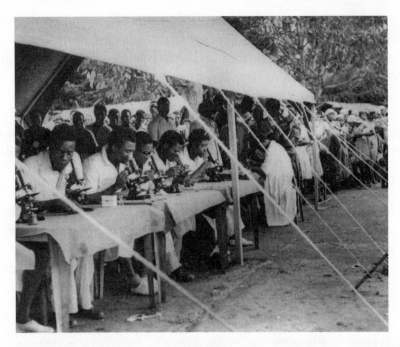

A Lomidinization campaign in Cameroon. Infocam, series *Visite d'un groupe mobile aux environs de Yaoundé,* "Examen des lames de sang au microscope," 1951 (151702-B). © Infocam.

in propaganda images, had already attained exceptional levels of efficacy, as measured in terms of populations covered and treated. According to its logic, the individualization of treatment was defined as dangerous and therefore was prohibited—for example, the accident in Bafia, Cameroon, in 1930 was blamed on the initiative taken by a doctor seeking to "adapt" the therapeutic dosage of tryparsamides to specific cases of sleeping sickness.[28] Individual or clinical approaches were thus reserved to the domain of research, to be practiced only in sites designated for experimentation, such as Ayos.[29] The utopia of standardized medicine, dreamed of by doctors in the metropole familiar with Fordist experiments, such as Dr. Destouches (Céline),[30] was in sleeping sickness control already within sight in the 1930s. Was there nothing new, then, in the practice of mass Lomidinization?

On the organizational level, there were obvious continuities. As before, the campaigns operated in the form of mobile tours lasting several days, relying on the same ritual of massively summoning populations to predefined points along the teams' routes, as well as on a steep hierarchy, in which a "European" doctor was entrusted with the supervision of several teams, each composed of a fleet of nurses and "coolies." For example, in 1952 in Cameroon, fewer than ten colonial doctors oversaw two hundred thousand annual injections of Lomidine and the testing of eight hundred thousand individuals by mobile teams.[31]

Yet, while it relied on an existing, well-oiled infrastructure, Lomidinization also disrupted the functioning of campaigns by introducing a new goal: to preventively treat every healthy subject. This put new pressure on the act of testing (the microscopic examination of a drop of blood). If trypanosome carriers were missed and thus treated as if healthy, that is, with only preventive injections, they would be exposed to the risk of developing "masked" infections, which were harder to treat.[32] True to the principle of prophylaxis, treatment was deemed to be a secondary task, one that was certainly necessary for the moment, but would not be for long. The microscopists trained to identify trypanosomes bore a heavy responsibility: to miss the fewest possible "positives" by giving time and attention to each slide, while at the same time hurrying to ensure that "negatives" proceeded to Lomidinization at a good pace. The number of microscopes used for testing was thus every campaign's limiting factor; among the iconic propaganda images were photographs of rows of microscopists at work.[33]

The most obviously novel element was the intramuscular injection of pentamidine, dosed at 4 milligrams per kilogram. A new workstation had to be inserted into the team's workflow and added to the circuit followed by patients through the mobile dispensary/laboratory—the *hangar médical* (medical shed), as it was called from the 1950s. A new column also appeared on the individual index cards distributed during campaigns. Lomidinization was placed at the end of the "therapeutic chain," after weighing and testing. Preparing and injecting the solution were technically demanding acts, particularly with respect to guaranteeing sterility; they formed a bottleneck in campaign operations.

Pentamidine injections thus heightened the demand for efficiency that was imposed on the chain as a whole; through this chain, it must not be forgotten, passed the *entirety* of the population visited. Rationalization was pushed to its highest degree—in some instructions, even the gestures of each hand were specified ("the operator, with his left hand, then seizes the stamp").[34] The best nurses were chosen as Lomidinizers.[35] Each step in the chain was timed, and the cadence of the injections was measured: it was estimated at the confer-

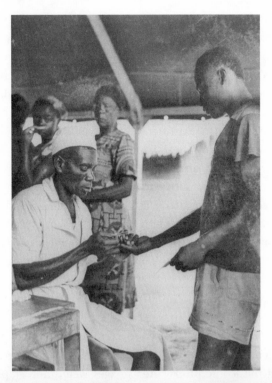

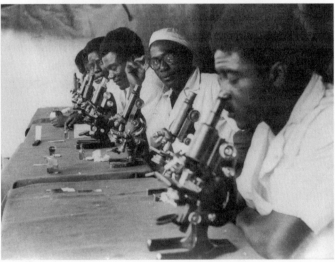

Taking blood samples and examining blood under the microscope. Infocam, series *Visite d'un groupe mobile aux environs de Yaoundé*, "Examen des lames de sang au microscope," 1951 (151702-C, 151702-E). © Infocam.

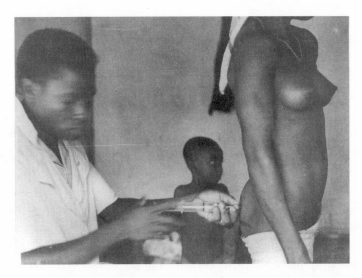

Intramuscular injection. The photo was erroneously given the legend "Lumbar puncture." This was likely a Lomidine injection. The presence of a partly naked young woman
is not surprising in the context of colonial propaganda, where the use of sexualized ico-
nography was frequent. Infocam, series *SHMP,* 1951 (151703–A). © Infocam.

ence in Brazzaville that "with a well-trained team we can perform about 500
preventive Lomidine injections per day."[36] Averages did often reach hundreds
of injections per day and per team; an oft-cited figure was three hundred per
morning (work ceased during the heat of the afternoon). Lotte, in AEF, noted:
"with trained personnel, we can inject 80 individuals per hour" (more than
one a minute).[37]

Injections of pentamidine solution were painful and irritating, and they
often caused edema. Even doctors recognized that it was hard to administer
a considerable volume (5–15 cubic centimeters) in the gluteal muscles. That
the "English" powder, which was more soluble, made it possible to halve the
volume of injected solution, elicited bitter remarks;[38] the organic ties binding
the French medical community to Spécia created an obligation, at the beginning, of fidelity to the "French" Lomidine salts at the cost of trickier and more
painful injection practices.[39] Nationalism had its price.

The importance given to resting was also new. The hypoglycemic and vagosympathetic effects of pentamidine—the very effects underlying its discovery
—could provoke problematic reactions following injection. Even at low prophylactic doses, adverse effects included fainting, vertigo, vomiting, and diarrhea

co-occurring with a sudden drop in arterial tension. These reactions, sometimes described as "states of shock," were reported from the very first trials
and never stopped being a cause for concern (even as they were downplayed
in publications).[40] Generally, the chosen solution was to require individuals
to fast before injection and to force them to rest, lying down, afterward; Jorge
Varanda found, in his research on Angola, extraordinary photographs of entire
villages lying flat on the ground.[41] Provisions for a resting space and post-
injection monitoring thus had to be integrated into the rational machine of
mass campaigns, even if this step, by its nature, eluded standardizing. Cardiac
tonics (adrenaline, camphorated oil) had to be available in case of fainting.
While adverse reactions were described in most articles as "rare and benign,"[42]
they nevertheless motivated additional experiments in search of a means to
prevent them; in Cameroon, Spécia arranged for tests of Lomidine in tablet
form and in combination with Moranyl, but the results were inconclusive.[43]
There were also trials of the administration of an antihistamine (Phénergan
produced by Spécia), then known to be effective in "states of shock," prior to
injection; the efficacy of this strategy was more convincing.[44]

Adverse effects left their imprint. Nurses still remember the dramatic effects
of Lomidine taken on a full stomach: those who lied about fasting suffered
for it.[45] For the doctors who orchestrated the campaigns, however, these were
technical problems and needed to be managed as such.

A Life-Size Experiment

"Chemoprophylaxis is still, too often, conducted haphazardly. Yet the value of
such a weapon depends entirely on how it is applied. Therefore, we will define
the technical, tactical and strategic principles on which realistic and rational
action can be based," explained Colonel-Doctor Lotte, the head of mobile
teams in AEF.[46] Pentamidinization went hand in hand with planning. The
function of the health services pyramid, of which the apex at the international
level was the BPITT, was not only to produce statistics, but also to centralize
expertise and decision making regarding the organization of campaigns.

Above all, we must consider this program as a "life-size experiment." This
is not a historian-imposed metaphor. Lotte himself vividly evoked this image
to describe the space across which campaigns were deployed: "AEF, because
of the size of its territory and the low density of its population, can be compared
to a huge petri dish in which the trypanic seed has been planted. [Its] colonies

can be studied separately. This particularity, while posing huge practical difficulties, is particularly favorable to the analysis of epidemiological factors."[47]

Even after trials had confirmed the efficacy of Lomidinization, the method continued to be conceptualized as an experiment. Careful monitoring of its results relied, for the first time in the history of sleeping sickness control, on statistical tests.[48] These shed new light on the epidemic as a whole and made it possible to forge new theoretical tools—not without a certain degree of fascination with mathematical elegance.[49] The epidemic as a whole—its natural history, its ecology, and even its individual physiological basis—was reinterpreted through the experiment of massive Lomidinization.

The metaphor of experimentation ordered the health services' practice: the precision of the results became a goal in itself. Campaign supervisors also insisted on the experimental significance of the presence rate. In Cameroon, for example, they congratulated themselves on a presence rate of 99 percent in the region of Yokadouma—not as a sign of a highly disciplined population, nor even because it guaranteed maximum efficacy, but rather because it "assured the reality" of the results.[50] In AEF, Lotte reiterated that "all efforts must be directed toward obtaining complete convocations. . . . At 100 [percent] of presence . . . the probability that the numerical results will be accurate and that their analysis will be justified is complete. At 50 [percent] of presence, this probability is one out of two. . . . This is no longer an experiment but a survey. . . . It is advisable to react and to do all in our power to respect, in the practical domain, the imperatives of the experimental method."[51]

This program thus contributed to the broader emergence of a form of experimental governmentality, by which development is approached as a large-scale scientific experiment.[52] Mass chemoprophylaxis came to be legitimated not only as a response to a public health emergency, but also in terms of its experimental value. Such a justification might, once epidemic threats subsided, prove more durable: an experiment, even if it results in failure, retains intrinsic value.

In line with this logic, the militarization of public health was pushed to its limits. In the French case, the hierarchy of mobile health services ensured the standardization of protocols, the circulation of information throughout the empire, smooth operations, and control over costs—yet this demanded considerable bureaucratic work. In the midst of the Indochina War, which mobilized many young colonial doctors, the promise of new drugs and hopes for eradication inspired an escalation—both practical and semantic—of references to military techniques. Because the new drug would be revolutionary only if it was accompanied by organizational change, some grew impatient. Lotte, for example, complained: "Our weapons have made remarkable progress, but our tactics have remained at the stage of the prophylactic middle ages of 1927. If Jamot were to return [from the dead], he would need only read the prospectus of a diamidine manufacturer to be perfectly up to date on the question and to get back to work at once."[53] The scale of the program, the systematic mapping of the epidemic, and the unprecedented opportunities for imperial and international integration encouraged the heads of health services to "think big," to think "strategy"—a term reiterated by every expert—and to put more emphasis on evaluating costs and results.[54] Doctors were also advised to keep their aims modest, in order to ensure they would be able to rigorously follow their given road maps.[55]

The martial metaphor was an inexhaustible source of inspiration. "The chief of a prophylaxis service must not [merely] be a functionary responsible for applying an administrative and technical routine. [He] is a general of operations who ponders his plans, reconnoiters the territory to sound out the enemy, targets his forces to crush [this enemy] and knows, when necessary, to change fronts,"[56] wrote Lotte with passion. The "general of operations . . . must also make the best use of the means at hand. If he cannot obtain the concentration [in means] of [the battles of] Verdun, la Malmaison or Garigliano, he can cover, with less artillery, the fronts that can thus be stabilized or attenuated, while waiting for the factories of the interior (that is, mass education and social progress) to provide him with abundant weapons and munitions," wrote Colonel-Doctor Masseguin on the basis of his experiences in AOF.[57] Doctors from Angola to Senegal, it seems, did not know how else to express themselves.

It is difficult to address such rhetorical excesses without indulgence or irony. This type of language was criticized even by contemporaries: "I don't much like this comparison with military technique" was handwritten into the margin of a report by a reader at the Ministère de la France d'Outre-Mer.[58] And yet, it seems important to take seriously the enthusiasm of animated doctors, especially young doctors, who found in such narratives a lexicon for imagining and describing their mission and their actions, that is, a technology of the self.[59] The doctors responsible for the most practical dimensions of the campaigns, those who worked as chiefs of teams or of regions, were often in their first post in Africa. This was the case for Jacques Pierre Ziegler, who went to AEF to put his thesis on chemoprophylaxis into practice by becoming the doctor in chief of an SGHMP sector in Chad.[60] For a doctor who was not yet thirty years old to direct a team and to elaborate a "tactic" was an opportunity to "be one's own [man]," part "king of the bush," part "boy scout of public health," as one of the doctors said.[61] In the same vein, Léon Lapeyssonnie, a spokesperson for this generation—and one of the first French doctors to use Lomidine—would later write: "And many of us found joy in watching as, before us, a project, a building, a new medical technique came into being, which would have taken twenty years in the metropole. It is intoxicating . . . to create, to bring a baby, an enterprise, into the world, when you are thirty years old."[62] As it was used and celebrated as "a weapon of total efficacy," Lomidinization also "galvanized the passion" of a generation of colonial doctors.[63]

The Time of Miracles

No matter where they came from—the Belgian Congo, AEF, Cameroon—the first results erased any lingering doubt. In most instances, the administration of a single injection of pentamidine to every member of an entire population resulted in a drastic drop in disease incidence. Never before had success in the fight against sleeping sickness come so quickly. The goal was no longer merely to control the epidemic; it was now to eradicate the disease. In the early 1950s, as cases of sleeping sickness grew rare across previously affected regions, eradication was the only reason left to keep deploying campaigns. In time, surely, "the curve [would follow a] tangent toward zero."[64]

A success story emerged at that time. It was generated largely by high-ranking doctors, those who kept their gaze fixed on the "vertical drop" of indicators,[65] and by end-of-career colonial figures. This story was, above all, a narrative of rupture with the past. The success of preventive pentamidine had upstaged the Jamot method and its equivalents, which were based on testing and treating the infected—mockingly called "hook and line fishing."[66] In Cameroon, sleeping sickness camps (*hypnoseries*), like the Centre Jamot in Yaoundé, were said to have become "vestiges of past battles"; the gathering of incurable patients was "a now obsolete formula [that] had made way for a more dynamic mode of action."[67] In the same vein, Dr. Chesterman had wondered aloud at the Royal Society in London, with reference to the practice of "clearing" in a discussion of tsetse fly control projects in northern Nigeria, whether it might not "somehow . . . belong to the pre-pentamidine era."[68] Doctors in Angola indulged in a similar daydream; here are their words, from a French translation of a report written in Portuguese: "We are convinced that, in 1956, the figures of table XXVIII [showing the progression of the epidemic in the late 1940s] will have the faded and moldy aspect of unpleasant things that have become history."[69]

The narrative of the success story was also one of miracles. In various colonial and tropical medicine journals, articles spoke of "wonder."[70] Propaganda services dispatched photographers on the ground, and, repeatings doctors' statements, reporters announced in 1949 the "quasi-certainty of stamping out, through chemical protection, a fearful tropical affliction for which there was no hope of a vaccine."[71] In the *Bulletin de la Société de Pathologie Exotique*, there was mention in 1951 of "absolute control over the trypanosomiasis endemic" in AEF.[72] In AOF that same year, Dr. Joseph Diallo hoped to "almost completely eliminate sleeping sickness."[73] Mobilizing the usual tropes of this kind of narrative, as old as colonial and missionary medicine—native ignorance to be surmounted, the courage of doctors, miracles obvious to all, the radiance of the nation and of science—other colonial doctors published their own accounts of the miracle, as in the following example from AEF: "The epidemic focus of Nola is being repopulated. The natives trust the 'new medicine.' They gather together, create new villages and expand the crops they were about to abandon to flee the plague. . . . The number of children between 0 and 1 year, that is of births, have tripled since chemoprophylaxis was implemented."[74]

In the same vein but adding a light patriotic touch, Dr. Henri Jonchère described the situation in AOF: "This method now enjoys . . . great popularity. The natives themselves solicit its application and [the doctor in chief of a sector] could even write: 'many Liberian subjects, when a team visited the canton of Manalaye [Guinea, AOF], crossed the border to obtain the benefits of this French enterprise.'"[75]

Drawing on a register common among trypanosomiasis experts, who rarely missed an opportunity to mention the sexual problems resulting from the disease, a self-congratulatory report remarked in 1952 that "chemoprophylaxis with Lomidine, after a period of abstention, [has conquered] its rightful place in the region of Man, where Lomidine has the reputation of making men virile and women fertile."[76] Indiscipline was no longer a threat to public health; now Lomidine itself disciplined populations: "By its effects, which are dazzling from the outset, it kindles great hope among populations. . . . The punctuality with which populations from the villages go, on the selected dates, to the sites of convocation is proof of this."[77]

In Angola, pentamidinization brigades were visited as if officials were attending a performance: the governor-general spent three days in the field in May 1950 and requested that a film be made on the topic. "Everything runs smoothly," wrote a journalist from the delegation.

> Everything in the team [has] a well-defined function; the schedule of activities is respected and everything is executed with a level of synchronicity that is awe inspiring. We were not, in Angola, used to seeing a task executed like this! From the moment the native enters the camp until the exit, every single step is noted, measured, controlled.[78]

The pentamidinization machine was an aesthetic experiment, sometimes compared to choreography or a "pantomime," some said with malice.[79] It would be inaccurate to reduce these descriptions to an artifact of propaganda—in eastern Cameroon, some elderly people can still imitate the sounds and dance-like movements of a screening operation. Here is more about the Portuguese version from 1950:

> With an admirable synchronicity and chronometric precision, without yelling or pushing, with an altogether remarkable discipline, the natives accepted and obeyed every prescription of the health agents. The reputation of Pentamidine has spread and reached every native tribe. To every site where, today, a sleeping sickness control team stops, billions of [N]egroes rush en masse, often from very far away and sometimes even from beyond borders. That "negroes" let themselves be impressed by [the] Brigades' way of proceeding is thus unsurprising: they came en masse to be examined and protected by "Pentamidine"—a word they saluted with "hurrahs" when we passed in our cars.[80]

Getting to Zero

Hardly five years after the campaigns had begun, the first announcements came of the "definitive concretization of this wonderful dream that our predecessors dared not contemplate: the eradication, in the historical land of 'sleep,' of the most devastating plague that ever ravaged tropical Africa."[81] In December 1953, the official journal of the colonial health corps, *Médecine Tropicale*, dedicated a special issue to trypanosomiasis, to broadcast the "great hope [that] was born, over the last ten years, with the introduction of diamidines in chemoprophylaxis."[82]

Filled with publicity inserts for Spécia products, the special issue provided an overview of Lomidinization campaigns across the Union française. Written by authorities from various colonies, each article was more enthusiastic than the last. Confidence in the new drug made doctors bold: a military psychiatrist with the rank of colonel, Pierre Gallais, reported trials of experimental inoculations of trypanosomiasis (!), which was then cured in all subjects with Lomidine.[83] In his introductory article, General-Doctor J. H. Raynal expressed the consensus by concluding that "it would take only a few more years of perseverance to relegate sleeping sickness in the black country to the status of a bad memory."[84] By late 1953, the time had come to ponder what had been accomplished: "one of the most magnificent public health victories of our civilization."[85]

French doctors unhesitatingly turned this victory into grounds for national pride. In theses, reports, and articles, the scientific story of the method's discovery by Launoy was stabilized.[86] The French tropicalist field as a whole approved of Lomidine, a "French product," which, they noted smugly, had displaced Pentamidine, the "English product" from May & Baker.[87] In 1951, Launoy, who liked to point out to readers that the vast Lomidinization programs were no more than implementations of his laboratory experiments, went off to see the miracles with his own eyes, "in this black Africa for which he had worked so much," as one of his biographers would say. He was welcomed in Bobo-Dioulasso by General-Doctor Jonchère, the head of the SGHMP in AOF, who would spend the end of his career working for Spécia. Launoy returned to Africa in 1952 and 1954, trips that were both scientific and social, and met with administrators, doctors, and local representatives of Spécia.[88]

In early 1954, one of the great veterans of "la trypano," Gaston Muraz, paid tribute to the method in an article published by a journal funded in part by Spécia: *L'Essor Médical dans l'Union Française* (The Rise of Medicine in the French Union), which was used as a platform by French colonial doctors in the 1950s. Titled, with the sobriety typical of Muraz's literary work, "Yes, Intertropical Africa Can and Must Cure Sleeping Sickness by Generalizing Lomidinization across All Contaminated Regions," the article—in which he cites Claude Bernard prominently—forgoes all nuance: "we have an *immediate obligation to create* chemically protected areas in all zones contaminated by human trypanosomiasis."[89] A few months later, Muraz wrote again in the same journal: "It will have taken fifty years of clinic[al medicine] and of chemotherapy to equip ourselves with *a veritably effective weapon, Lomidinization* with which, at once, we will work resolutely in French black Africa toward the eradication of human trypanosomiasis."[90]

On December 21, 1954, Gaston Muraz spoke to the Académie nationale de

OUI, L'AFRIQUE INTERTROPICALE
PEUT ET DOIT GUÉRIR DE

LA MALADIE DU SOMMEIL

EN GÉNÉRALISANT

LA LOMIDINISATION

DE TOUTES SES RÉGIONS CONTAMINÉES

Par G. MURAZ
Médecin Général Inspecteur du Corps de Santé colonial
(C.R.)

L'ÉRADICATION

de la

MALADIE DU SOMMEIL

par la

LOMIDINISATION

Par G. MURAZ
Médecin Général Inspecteur du
Corps de Santé coloniol (C.R.)

Gaston Muraz, *L'Essor Médical dans l'Union Française 3* (1954), 15, and 4 (1954), 45.

médecine to praise the "very wide[ly applied] measures of intramuscular injection of aromatic diamidines (Lomidine) already implemented over the past few years, which strive for the eradication of sleeping sickness": "Once again, I declare, straight out, that Lomidinization is still a *great medicosocial victory* in which overseas French medicine, by its fertile demographic consequences for this underpopulated Africa, has taken the largest share [of responsibility]. It will have knocked out the epidemic 'genius' of one of the most serious afflictions, of which the end result is depopulation after slow death."[91]

Pentamidine's victories were also celebrated on the other side of the channel where, with typical British understatement, the "weapon's power" was recognized,[92] yet the prospect of eradication remained in doubt. Doctors in Brussels archived a copy of an article written in January 1948 by a special correspondent of the *New York Herald Tribune* who had visited Léopoldville, "Africa Is Winning Its Battle against Sleeping Sickness." The article quotes Dr. Thomas, the head of the health services in the Belgian Congo: "If current progress continues, sleeping sickness will be virtually eliminated from the population of the Congo over the next 10 to 20 years," thanks to "a sufficiently cheap and abundantly available drug for use as large-scale prophylaxis."[93]

One last anecdote: In 1952, a debate arose among the French, Belgians, British, and Portuguese who had gathered for a conference in Lourenço Marques (now Maputo), Mozambique, on the subject of a novel problem arising in the wake of pentamidine's success. The color codes for mapping the epidemic on a continental scale, which had been defined in 1948, needed to be completely amended. "The representation of the map, with the colours internationally adopted, of the indexes of circulating virus, obtained after the first pentamidinization, looses [*sic*] all interest, the sky blue being the only used colour."[94] According to the code, sky blue represented rates under 1 percent. The new code, delegates proposed, needed to adopt a revised, more appropriate scale, using a range of colors to represent rates lower than 0.1, 0.2, and 0.3 percent. Africa was recolored—in shades of zero.

In any case, this discovery of long-term chemical protection against trypano-somiasis is certainly the greatest entitlement to the gratitude of humanity obtained by Léon Launoy. All those who have been involved, closely or from a distance, with the major tropical endemics will agree that, for psychological reasons, it is very difficult to obtain, from primitive populations, trust in therapeutic methods requiring long-term treatment: if, after a single medical consultation, the patent is not cured . . . the vil-lage witch doctor persuades him that he was wrong to trust the white doctor, [who] is powerless. If, however, we instead [dispense] long-acting drugs, which can, with a single injection or a single oral administration, provide definitive cure or immunity, the prestige of Western medicine [will be] total, and mass success [will be] obtainable. . . . In his work, Léon Launoy was thus a precursor who set chemotherapeutic research in tropical disease on the path which [turns out to have been] the path of the future.

Pr. M. Guillot, member of the Académie de pharmacie and the Académie nationale de médecine, in a brochure (circa 1972) published by Spécia laboratories in homage to their former scientific director, Professor Léon Launoy, 17.

CHAPTER FIVE

Lomidine, the Individual, and Race

In countries where everything is scarce, the doctor is forced to put the prevention of epidemics above the relief of individual suffering. Above all, save the race; this, in most cases, is the key directive.[1]

In 1951, in an article published by the Parisian *La Semaine des Hôpitaux* (*Hospitals Weekly*), Dr. Louis-Paul Aujoulat, the secretary of state of Overseas France, reiterated the basic postulate underlying health policy in colonial Africa: priority should be given to interventions at the scale of the social body—"the race"—rather than at the individual scale. Although Aujoulat was a Catholic missionary doctor and usually rather reticent on the topic of methods of mass hygiene, this statement reveals the extent to which "medicine for the race" was by the postwar years a common denominator of colonial public health. "To preserve and treat not individuals but the mass": this motto of the social hygiene plan of the Brazzaville Conference of 1944 seems to align perfectly with sleeping sickness prophylaxis campaigns. Their methods were conceptualized, practiced, and evaluated at the scale of populations.

Yet pentamidinization was not merely an instantiation of this collective vision of public health—if so, it would not make for a particularly original case. On the contrary, preventive pentamidine, at least initially, destabilized the mass hygiene model: first, because it was addressed to healthy individuals but also, more important, because it induced unanticipated effects that puzzled doctors. The history of pentamidinization is also a history of the problems it posed as experts sought to understand its mode of action and to explain an efficacy that was prodigious yet erratic. In this chapter I trace how doctors understood and surmounted technical issues posed by the drug, which ranged from side effects (which were sometimes fatal) to its inability to protect some individuals.

Because of its unpredictable effects, its agency,[2] pentamidine demanded considerable theoretical work in order to remain trustworthy. This work, which took up much of the content of scientific publications on the topic, led paradoxically to a reaffirmation of the hygienist principles that had seemed to be undermined by the new method. Preventive pentamidine thus stimulated the emergence of a reinforced version of "medicine for the race," which was understood in a double sense: first, as a population-level medicine, with its collective rationality and practices, and second, as a racialized medicine, which used and consolidated the perceived racial differences between Europeans and Africans. Compulsory for African collectives yet too dangerous for European individuals, pentamidine became a racialized drug. The sole consequence of its dramatically uncertain effects at the individual scale, which were recognized as unpredictable from the very first campaigns, was to strengthen doctors' confidence in the method and encourage them in recommending even greater zeal in its implementation.

Colonial doctors' enthusiasm about the imminent eradication of trypanosomiasis in 1954, after six years of great announcements and great operations, can be understood as a way of patching the cracks that had been slowly fissuring the theoretical and practical edifice of chemoprophylaxis. In other words, invoking eradication was not a precondition for the implementation of Lomidinization, but instead a way of resolving its inability to work as chemical protection at the individual level.

The Ambiguities of Chemoprophylaxis

The first problem colonial doctors encountered was a theoretical one: What, exactly, is "chemoprophylaxis"? On the surface, the answer was simple: chemoprophylaxis was a new approach to controlling sleeping sickness, developed in animals by Professor Léon Launoy and then implemented in humans on a large scale. Its basis was the chemical protection of healthy individuals against potential infection by trypanosomes,which had been demonstrated in various animal models by the Spécia expert.[3] Such a definition located the method within a basic scientific tradition, that of the prestigious Laboratoire de prophylaxie chimique (Laboratory of Chemical Prophylaxis) of the Faculté de Paris. References to the Parisian scientist Launoy—the "precursor"[4]—added a touch of distinction to articles on the topic, which systematically restated Launoy's definition of chemical prophylaxis based on an explicit link between pentamidine and vaccination: "One must understand [chemical prophylaxis] as the use of a method which, by introducing in the healthy organism a relatively small quantity of a given chemical product, provokes in this organism a state of resistance such that this organism is protected, during many months, against a determined condition."[5]

Yet recourse to this biological-experimental definition was also expedient and retrospective. The genealogy of pentamidinization leads to a history that is messier—and also more colonial.

Indeed, from the beginning of the twentieth century, the dominant model for colonial public health was "social prophylaxis," which entailed treating the virus reservoir, a collective entity made up of carriers of infectious pathogens, to achieve a preventive (prophylactic) effect at the population level. Applied in Europe for the control of tuberculosis and venereal disease (the term used at the time was "social hygiene"), this model originated in a colonial context as the German bacteriologist Robert Koch experimented with what would be called the "Koch method" beginning in 1897.[6] The method was first used on a large scale by German colonial doctors to control malaria in the city of Dar es Salaam; in 1901, they attempted to detect and to treat with quinine every single individual carrier of the parasite. By shrinking the virus reservoir in this way, the hope was to control, or even eradicate, malaria: treating individuals functioned as collective prevention.[7] Little did it matter that they did not succeed: the German experiment in Dar es Salaam became in the early twentieth century a key model for German, French, and Belgian colonial doctors, who transposed its principles to sleeping sickness. Rarely in the history of public health has a failure been so successful: references to the model were omnipresent from the Mission permanente de prophylaxie de la maladie du sommeil (Permanent Mission for Sleeping Sickness Prophylaxis), created by Eugène Jamot in 1926, to the mobile hygiene and prophylaxis services of the 1940s, even though these campaigns did not actually use a preventive method, strictly defined. A young doctor who had just arrived in Africa said: "It was the social body as [a] fragment of a whole that I was to work with; it was the community that I had to protect and to defend against disease."[8] Social prophylaxis was the lingua franca of colonial doctors.

Given the predominance of this view, which blurred the line between prevention and therapy and which envisaged the possibility of an "African individual" only in the relatively distant future, it is difficult to distinguish the novelty—even though it was radical—of preventive pentamidine. This may be why historians have paid so little attention to the technique. The method also inherited a legacy of ambiguities.

The very term "pentamidinization" (and Lomidinization) echoed the neologism "quininization" (*Chinisierung*) used by German doctors earlier in the century to refer to the test-and-treat program of Dar es Salaam. This first neologism conflated treatment and prevention, being used to designate both the indiscriminate treatment of "natives," defined as a virus reservoir, *and* the consumption of preventive quinine by healthy Europeans, for whom it was a long-standing daily ritual.[9] In the field of sleeping sickness, neologisms such as "atoxylation" and "Bayerization" were cast from the same mold in the 1920s–30s to designate either a form of chemoprophylaxis (for example, the use of Bayer 205 in the Belgian Congo) or the indiscriminate treatment of the populations of high prevalence regions (applied to all people, without testing).[10] It would be a mistake to look for retrospective clarification of these definitions: at the time, chemoprophylaxis was understood within a fluid distinction between prevention and treatment, which partly overlapped with a racial distinction between European individuals and African collectives.

The adoption of preventive pentamidine was thus rooted in ambiguity; it was a means both of protecting healthy subjects by injecting a whole population and of protecting healthy individuals by each personal injection.

The Drug That Was Too Effective

A second problem arose as the earliest experiments unfolded. The effects of pentamidinization at the epidemiological level were extraordinarily rapid. What might explain this? What biological mechanism could give rise to such a "miracle"? The physiological interpretation of protection was a tricky matter. As the young expert Ziegler wrote tersely in 1948, "The explanation of the mechanism of the prevention of trypanosomiasis by diamidines has not yet been demonstrated."[11]

The available experimental data were still tenuous and based on animals. The existence of direct action on the parasite through interference with glucose metabolism was unproblematic. There was, however, little additional information to support any conclusions beyond this. Doctors could only hypothesize; they hesitated between the possibility of an "immunizing" effect—supposing that pentamidine might stimulate the organisms' own defenses in the long term—and that of a purely chemical mode of action, which supposed that pentamidine "waited" for the parasite inside the organism.

The stake of these debates was eminently practical: the question of how long protection lasted was a critical one, for it dictated, in theory, the timing of campaigns (and therefore their cost). As a French doctor explained in Brazzaville in 1948, ideally it would be possible to determine the "maximal subtoxic concentration . . . that could confer protection lasting one or two years," so as not to "disturb the populations too often."[12] The Belgian experiments on "volunteers" in Léopoldville had suggested that protection lasted about six months. This time span was confirmed by the first trials; new infections were rarely detected during the first year after injection. This supported the official recommendation to repeat injections every six months—even while colonial doctors and authorities acknowledged that the matter was still awaiting "research . . . to give more precise information on the nature and duration of the protective action of diamidines."[13] Yet pentamidinization, as it was implemented on a massive scale after 1948, did not maintain this rhythm. Campaigns were conducted annually, or even only every two years, in some cases intentionally so as not to wear out populations' tolerance for the injections.[14] Surprisingly, the results were, as a general rule, just as good, which was almost embarrassing. Could it be that Lomidine protected for several years? Few authors even attempted to interpret the results.

How could such long protection times be explained? On the pharmacological front, there were no data on which to base an answer.[15] There was agreement that pentamidine was active at very low concentrations and that, following a phase of rapid urinary elimination, it was stocked in tissues and gradually diffused into the plasma; this is what accounted for its long-lasting effects. Yet the details remained vague; it was suggested, for example, that pentamidine, in order to act durably, would have to "bind to large plasmatic molecules" or not "pass through the renal filter."[16] The problem was not limited to the question of the duration of protection. On the epidemiological front, the sudden drop in disease incidence, often after just a single campaign, was also puzzling. By 1948, it was already clear that pentamidine's mode of action could not be understood at the scale of the individual only. Delegates at the conference in Brazzaville were surprised to discover the results of the first trial in AEF: "Lieutenant-Colonel-Doctor Beaudiment . . . remarked that it seemed strange to note not only the absence of [trypanosome-infected individuals found by] control [tests] in injected subjects, but also among controls. The chairman answered that indeed this observation had not escaped him and that this result, also recorded elsewhere, could seem paradoxical and inconclusive with regard to the efficacy of protection by diamidines."[17]

The outcome clearly "exceeded expectations": in the trials, Lomidinization even protected control subjects who had not received the injection! The explanations put forward in Brazzaville for this result were not self-evident. Colonel-Doctor Saleun, the session's chairman, first pointed to the efficacy of screening tests and the prior treatment of infected persons, which led to "a notable decrease in the virus reservoir," and of "agronomic prophylaxis measures."[18] In other words, he did not credit chemoprophylaxis per se. However, Saleun, who was directly responsible for the trials in question, also proposed as "just hypotheses" the "possibility of the destruction of [trypanosomes] in the glossina who feed on pentamidinized subjects" or of a "reduction in the infecting power of the vector" associated with the prophylactic injection.[19] Until the end of the 1950s, the action of pentamidine on tsetse flies (called, esoterically, the trypanosome's "extrinsic cycle") remained a mystery. Experiments were initiated to determine the possibility that infected glossinas were "sterilized" (in the infectious sense) by a blood meal taken from preventively treated patients, but the results were unclear.[20] Still, this hypothesis long continued to circulate among doctors: tsetse flies Lomidinize themselves by biting Lomidinized individuals.

Despite these uncertainties, there emerged an understanding of pentamidine's action at the level of the parasitic cycle, encompassing humans and flies: this theory suggested that a momentary yet complete interruption in transmission, rather than long-lasting protection, might be the cause of the slump in the epidemic.[21] This hypothesis was rather complicated since it required a dynamic model of the epidemic, but it solved the enigma of pentamidine's collective benefits. Doubts about the method thus stimulated a new epidemiology of sleeping sickness that was centered on the "trypanosome-human-fly cycle,"[22] departing from prior, more static representations (a virus reservoir and a vector as alternative targets). Such doubts also informed new control strategies, namely, an intensification of campaigns, which should be deployed with "implacable rigor."[23] A decisive strike was needed to "interrupt, once and for all, the perpetuation [of the] cycle."[24]

As the initial surprise wore off, the collective effects of Lomidine were recorded on a regular basis and even scientifically quantified: "in a well-defined region, . . . the Lomidinization of ⁵⁄₇ of the population reduces by a factor of six the infestation rate of this population as a whole."[25] The discovery that individual protection led to collective benefits was not, in itself, new to colonial sanitarians,[26] and they would later use the term "herd immunity," borrowed from veterinary science. Yet Lomidinization provided an opportunity to demonstrate this phenomenon on a statistical basis; it was compared to observations of smallpox vaccination, in which "vaccinating three quarters of the community can, for the most part, protect the remaining quarter."[27] In this way, the new method was connected back to the old model of social prophylaxis, and it fit more clearly within the dominant paradigm of colonial medicine.

The collective interpretation of chemoprophylaxis was also expedient, given how difficult it was to confirm and to explain its preventive effects at the scale of the individual. In 1954, after several thousand injections, only Van Hoof's experiments on the individuals Moya and Bonkumu provided any basis for the evaluation of pentamidine's preventive effects in humans at the level of individuals; the long-lasting magic bullet's mode of action remained unknown. However, the authority of the numbers obtained at the scale of whole regions brought closure to the debate: "The hypothesis of the prophylactic effect of the diamidines can now be elevated to a statistical law," affirmed Lotte in 1953.[28] And so, the first set of uncertainties about how to account for the power of the molecule was resolved. However, another, more awkward issue arose: What were Lomidinization's risks and benefits at the individual level?

Failures of Protection

Sometimes, pentamidine did not protect individuals. In some cases, trypanosome infections were diagnosed barely a few months after injection. How could these failures be explained?

Cases of trypanosomiasis in Lomidinized subjects were reported beginning in the first campaigns. Most of these people had already reached the "nervous" phase of the disease, presenting with signs of invasion of the cerebrospinal fluid. An interpretation was at hand: these were cases of already-infected individuals who had eluded diagnosis and for whom "the single injection was unable to stop the progression of the disease."[29] Blame was placed on nurse-microscopists and their lack of vigilance. Still, Lotte did take the trouble to measure the minimal frequency of testing errors; he arranged for a single group to be examined repeatedly and found that only 30 percent of infected subjects were accurately detected! A large proportion of the "contaminated protected" was thus "to be attributed to the failures of testing, not of chemoprophylaxis."[30] Some cases of what was called "apparent failure," however, concerned infections that appeared to be recent, suggesting that contamination had occurred soon after injection. Again, authors agreed not to blame "these failures . . . [on] chemoprophylaxis." One sector's doctor in chief identified as their cause an "organization of monitoring . . . not yet perfected. . . .

Some subjects [managed] to escape between the moment [of registration] and the moment when they were to be injected."[31]

Twenty-five Lomidinized and infected individuals were found in another sector in AEF. Yet the head of this campaign reported: "Experience . . . tells us that these 25 cases are not all failures. Operating in a dance hall of the village, which had hidden and numerous entrances, made it impossible to effectively control [people, many of whom,] after being examined and weighed, managed to escape the last act in the operation. Among these 25 [newly infected], the majority were clerks, employees, houseboys."[32] These seemingly innocuous sentences sketched out a new social pathology—the colonial disorder that was emerging in the 1950s—thwarting the all-powerful Lomidinization. Here, there was a village on the way to becoming an urban center, a dance hall environment foiling any possibility of control, and "natives" no doubt contaminated because they were neither villagers nor really "evolved," but instead in the pathological in-between state of clerks, employees, and houseboys. The pathologization of these new figures, perceived as the products of an out-of-control modernization, featured regularly in the contemporary medical literature; in its psychological variant, it was even mobilized in Kenya, for example, as a scientific explanation for anticolonial movements.[33] Individual indiscipline, namely the capacity to elude injection, accounted for individual failures. This explanation allowed for a reaffirmation of belief in the technique. Thus, an instability peculiar to Lomidinization reinforced colonial doctors' theoretical and sociological assumptions.

The same pattern—beginning with an observation of failure, ending with doctors' strengthened determination—occurred at the level of campaign planning. How could the difficulty of completely eradicating the disease be explained and surmounted? The question emerged in 1950, when campaigns, after years of effective pentamidinization, continued to come up against sporadic cases of infection. In the Belgian Congo, a new experimental approach by the FOREAMI in Kasai was adopted. It consisted in extending the space of protection into buffer zones: disease-free areas surrounding endemic focuses already under pentamidinization.[34] A new level of collectivization was reached when populations not even exposed to the risk of infection were targeted in the name of eradicating a neighboring epidemic focus. Thus, the limits of pentamidinization once again revitalized doctors' ambitions: if the technique did not work perfectly, surely this was because it was not being used on a large enough scale.

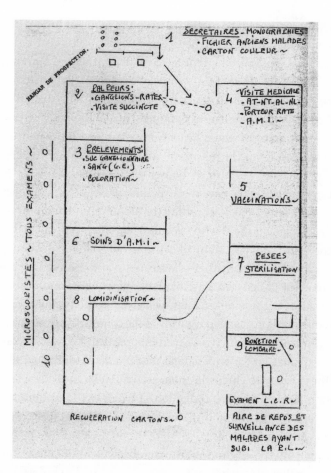

Organization of a medical screening hangar. Lomidinization was the last step in patients' circuit, after which they received an individual index card. F. Gauthier, *Lutte contre la trypanosomiase et la lèpre en Afrique* 1953–1960 (Éditions des Écrivains, Paris, 2000), 84.

Lomidinization Accidents: Accusing the Individual

Experts reached consensus on the cause of Lomidinization accidents—the accepted term for a range of conditions, including death, that occurred following injections. Debates about the method's safety were turned into an opportunity to reaffirm its value; problems were blamed on the carelessness or the indiscipline of "natives"—a category conflating nurses and patients. Once again, the figure of the pathological individual was invoked to explain the method's shortcomings and to justify the hardening and intensification of campaigns.

One type of accident was not specific to the new molecule; rather, it was caused by its mode of administration: local infections could develop at the injection site and could even progress to deadly cases of gangrene. A cause was close at hand: the "natives" themselves, of course. Responding to a series of fatal accidents resulting from post-injection abscesses, Gaston Muraz explained in 1954: "How, indeed, are we not to suffer a few failures of this highly preventive method . . . when careful investigations . . . inform us that the natives sometimes apply on the top part of their buttocks, site of the i/m [intramuscular] injection of Lomidine, 'plasters made of mud or of mashed banana.' "[35]

This comment merely added to an existing repertoire of harmful customs compiled by doctors, yet the issue it raised *was* a source of concern. An anonymous report, written circa 1953, expressed worry about the consequences of "a few septic accidents, infinitely rare considering the mass of injections administered, furthermore usually attributable to natives themselves but which risk discrediting such a perfect method."[36] It should be reiterated that, although always underplayed in official reports and publications, the issue of ensuring that injections were aseptic had preoccupied sleeping sickness doctors since the interwar years; in circular after circular, they relentlessly called team supervisors and nurses to order.[37] Other types of accident also were linked to injections, notably sciatic nerve damage, a typical consequence of improperly placed intramuscular injections. The same explanations were given: nurses' mistakes and the "apprehension and indocility of patients."[38] The irritating quality of pentamidine and the risks arising from the fast pace of the injections were never considered.

In addition, pentamidine posed specific problems of drug toxicity, which at the time were attributed to its hypoglycemic action. Although mentioned only as minor incidents in publications, these effects were worrying enough for authorities at the highest levels of the health services to launch investigations and for Spécia to arrange for trials to be conducted.[39] Compared to the analysis of other types of adverse effects, the interpretations of toxic accidents were more original and more scientific.

Cameroon served as a laboratory. In late 1954, Raymond Beaudiment, the head of the SHMP, and his two deputies devoted an entire report to the topic of Lomidinization accidents, which also described the series of trials, conducted with Spécia's advice, to identify a means of "preventing" this toxicity. The year 1953, they said, had seen an upsurge in "clinical complaints."[40] Problems arose in 20 percent of injections—two hundred thousand had been administered— and one death had been reported. The geographical distribution of the accidents was especially troubling. While some zones appeared to be "safe," others were at high risk. The cities of Nkongsamba and Douala and their outskirts, for example, had seen hundreds of cases of loss of consciousness. In explaining these disparities, Beaudiment ruled out the possibility of technical error since, in all cases, operations were performed "under the surveillance of a doctor and of an experienced health assistant." Learning of another cluster of incidents near Yaoundé, Beaudiment proposed a more elaborate hypothesis:

> The occurrence of accidents in the area of Yaoundé . . . confirms our *hypothesis of a vagosympathetic*[41] *instability peculiar to the residents of large [urban] centers* or of large commercial centers. It appears . . . to result, at the time of injection, in:
>
> - a factor of fearfulness and emotionality which is greater in these populations
> - the consumption of food in spite of prescriptions, [which is the] expression of a state of mind less inclined toward discipline
> - the abusive consumption of alcoholic beverages, of which the use increases extraordinarily upon coming into contact with large centers.[42]

Addressing accidents as an experimental fact led to the incrimination of an implicitly feminine "native" weakness. The taxonomy was scientific, thus providing experimental substance to a pathologization of urban residents and their disordered evolution that was prevalent in contemporary health reports. Indiscipline, already blamed as a cause of absenteeism, which impeded social prophylaxis, was now said to expose individuals themselves to the risk of accidents.

Cameroon's SHMP did not stop at the description of childish "natives." With support from Spécia, the service also sought to prevent accidents by experimenting in 1953–54 with new Lomidine preparations. First the doctors tried a gel solution that, by producing a "delayed effect," might reduce the shock of injection. Although the first results were promising, the trial was a failure: another death and two serious cases of cardiac complaints occurred in Douala. The SHMP then experimented with a new compound received from Spécia, a combination of Lomidine and Moranyl (the French equivalent of Bayer 205) called 4891 RP. The hope was that this compound would offer longer-lasting prophylactic protection and reduce the likelihood of accidents. Moranyl had been shown in animals, and then in human trials in Cameroon, to produce an antagonistic effect—Beaudiment spoke of a "buffer effect"—on some of Lomidine's adverse effects, such as loss of consciousness. A preliminary trial was considered to be successful despite "less [than] perfect tolerance from the local perspective"[43]—which presented as painful edema in the buttocks. Trials were extended to villages near Yaoundé, but unfortunately new problems of swelling and abscesses in the buttocks arose, forcing the suspension of the injections.

With no other answer at hand, the SHMP recommended a "provisional solution," "urging [its teams] to systematically precede the injection of Lomidine with an intravenous injection of Moranyl." The disadvantage of this attempt at technical innovation was that it would "slow the pace of Lomidinization"— surely an understatement given how burdensome this new procedure was (it entailed administering an intramuscular *and* an intravenous injection to the *entire* population). Still, its implementation allowed for operations to proceed "without any, not even minor, trouble across the entire territory"[44]—that is, except on one occasion signaled by Beaudiment: "Near Douala and Yaoundé, . . . on a first set of 163 coupled injections, 7 [cases of] indisposition with vomiting were recorded after just the injection of Moranyl, and despite this injection one serious [case of] syncope and the death of a 50 year old woman are to be deplored. The autopsy that was conducted did not, however, reveal any specific phenomenon except for the recent consumption of a medium-size meal."

There were enough complaints to put pressure on the SHMP to momentarily suspend Lomidinization in the area surrounding both cities. Beaudiment once again led the investigation, dismissed the possibility that the specific batch of Lomidine used was particularly toxic, and concluded with an irrefutable explanation of his series of experiments: "As we set out above and until more ample [*sic*] informed, we thus attribute these complaints to the vagosympathetic instability characteristic of certain populations."[45]

The experimental trajectory that Beaudiment and his deputies traced from one accident to another reveals rather tragically the lack of any formulation of the risks and benefits at the individual scale; the accidents were subsequently inverted to pathologize Africans and their responses. Even when it became imperative to stop campaigns that were doing harm, an overly emotional population was blamed. Once again, unexpected events brought doctors back into familiar territory.

Risks and Benefits

It might be objected that my analysis overstates doctors' awareness of the issues posed by the drug; that incoherence becomes apparent only in retrospect, as the product of an anachronistic transposition of our current ethical norms. Instead, it might be suggested, one should somehow take into account the spirit of the times, which would have rendered any pragmatic discussion of the method's value impossible. Yet several clues suggest that the contradictions peculiar to preventive pentamidine—which was simultaneously too effective and not effective enough, both dangerous and absolutely safe—were indeed perceived and expressed in these terms at the time. In other words, doctors were fully aware of these contradictions as they set out to resolve them.

Doubts about the method emerged from the outset and were explicitly formulated in terms of individual risks and benefits. Jacques Pierre Ziegler, a young expert on the method, admitted as early as 1948 that there were "still many skeptics. Some do not want to admit to the existence of [a] chemo-prophyla[ctic effect], others think the method has more drawbacks than advantages, or that we have no right to expose a healthy individual to the risk of an accident that might be deadly, since, if he [developed sleeping sickness] we could, in the majority of cases, cure him."[46] In Angola, colonists mocked the new method, calling it the *pentamentira* (a combination of the words for "pentamidine" and "lie," in the sense of falsehood or deception).[47]

Because it was applied to healthy individuals, chemoprophylaxis posed the problem of drug toxicity in novel terms. The toxicity of trypanosomiasis drugs had, with rare exceptions such as the incident of Bafia in Cameroon,[48] been accounted for in doctors' calculations either as a lesser evil, given the desperate prognosis of patients in advanced phases of the disease, or as the price to pay to "sterilize" patients,[49] that is, to render them noncontagious (but not necessarily to cure them). The use of preventive methods that exposed healthy subjects to risk made the issue of toxicity more sensitive, which was why the French and British remained cautious during the interwar period. But it was because pentamidine reduced the risk of accidents relative to other prophylactic drugs, such as Bayer 205 and propamidine, that it was considered to be more acceptable. Although Bayer 205 was used on a massive scale by Belgians, the drug provoked serious accidents, even cases of sudden death, while only providing incomplete protection. While Belgians persisted in finding that "the advantages of the method [when] used in heavily infested regions [prevailed] over its drawbacks,"[50] a British doctor instead judged in 1945 that "there seems no justification for compelling a health labourer to take this risk," thus condemning Bayerization.[51] Despite this, at the time of its first trials in 1946–48, pentamidine seemed to favorably rebalance the risk-benefit-cost equation. Doctors were not blinded by nor entrapped in standards of action that we today would find strange. Bypassing discussions of preventive pentamidine's risks and benefits at an individual level arose from rational deliberations.

A notable exception was the case of the British health services, whose personnel did not share the general enthusiasm for mass pentamidinization. The British sought to be pragmatic, aiming to tread carefully with the population and to save resources for fly control. The real burden of the epidemic, calculated proportionally to spending on control programs, was thus more influential than the prospect of eradication. Indeed, pentamidinization was implemented only selectively in Nigeria and in Sierra Leone, targeting small at-risk populations, such as miners. Yet at the international level, the debate was never polarized into a confrontation between two strategies; some in the British medical community envied the ambitiousness of French programs, regretting that "economic considerations govern the pace and extent of one's humanity."[52] Although the tone of the comparisons remained cordial, these diverging views reinforced an image of "Latins" (the category included the Belgians) being under the affective spell of Lomidinization.[53] In 1971, an English doctor was amused in a debate on the history of trypanosomiasis to find that he was the only defender of chemoprophylaxis in the room—"a rather rare quality in a Brit."[54]

A Racial Equation: The Case of Europeans

Must Europeans (referring to White people or colonists in 1950s Africa) submit to Lomidinization? This was not an entirely marginal question, given that some urban zones targeted by Lomidinization, such as Yaoundé, Bamako, and Léopoldville, were inhabited by thousands of colonists. Official publications did not even raise the issue. Following the logic of social prophylaxis, they recommended Lomidinization for all, implicitly including Europeans: "The method applies to all subjects; within a collectivity, there should be no discrimination."[55] In 1951, an overview of campaigns in AOF specifically stated that "on the whole, *in Europeans as well as in Africans*, the intramuscular injection of Lomidine is very well tolerated."[56] Documents aimed at local populations for propaganda purposes were equally explicit on this point: "Don't think that Lomidinization is reserved only to Africans! Europeans whose job it is to be in the bush, or those who live in the big centers and go, on Sundays, to fish in the ponds, the marshes, the rivers, or to hunt in the forest, are also warned of the risk they run, and are strongly encouraged to have themselves Lomidinized. Many request it spontaneously."[57]

Yet other sources, those oriented directly toward medical practitioners, proffered a different discourse; one might even say that their rhetorical efforts revealed, in their attempts to do the opposite, how thorny an issue this was. Manuals of tropical medicine, although written by the very same colonial doctors, were cautious about the value of giving Lomidine to Europeans. "Individual preventive injections . . . are to be reserved to Europeans who are particularly exposed because of their professional role," specified Vaucel, the author of a chapter on trypanosomiasis written with advice from several veterans of Lomidinization campaigns.[58] An official circular of the SGHMP in AOF was even more unequivocal: Lomidine was not recommended for Europeans. If, however, they insisted on it, numerous precautions would have to be taken—precautions, one might point out, that were hardly compatible with the rhythms of mass campaigns and that were not required for African recipients.

CHEMO-PROPHYLAXIS IN EUROPEANS

Whether at the request of an individual or of a group, the injection of diamidines in Europeans must <u>always be</u> administered by the <u>Sector Doctor-in-Chief.</u> After chemical and bacteriological examination of the subject, and determination that he is free of trypanosomiasis.

1. ensure that he is <u>willing (written declaration of the subject)</u>
2. <u>in-depth</u> medical examination:

from the cardiac point of view: auscultation, <u>tension</u>
from the <u>hepatorenal</u> point of view: antecedents, <u>albuminuria</u>.
Exclude from experimentation any subject with hypotension, anemia, hepatorenal antecedents or complications (liver abscess, nephritis with albuminuria, etc.).
Exclude any subject in the acute phase of a condition or whose general state is poor, or too old (over 50).[59]

These official instructions were confidential but crystal clear: for Europeans, Lomidine was dangerous and painful, while for Africans—including infants, pregnant women, and older adults (except when their general state was too poor)—it was compulsory.

In practice, the issue of Lomidinization in Europeans arose fairly frequently. Indeed, Spécia's advertising efforts and the colonial propaganda apparatus succeeded in drawing attention in both the metropole and African capitals to the availability of a "vaccination against sleeping sickness"—a conflation that was systematically suggested and perpetuated by specialists such as Launoy. Lomidine attracted a lot of attention; the disease was still widely feared, and the number of travelers to Africa was growing as the first regular airline routes were opened. Experts were solicited for advice. In France, the Institut Pasteur received the bulk of requests from private firms and public agencies that were concerned about their staffs. After deliberating with experts from the Ministère de la France d'Outre-Mer, the mother house issued instructions for transmission to the institutes in the colonies, which were in charge of managing individual Lomidinization requests locally. Thus, in 1950, Noël Bernard of the Institut Pasteur in Paris wrote to the director of the Dakar branch:

My dear Colleague,

The incidence of several cases of sleeping sickness among the staff of various private administrations has prompted their Parisian headquarters to put in a request for protection (they say vaccination) against this African endemic. Their wish is to treat their agents without any distinction among them.

Upon the advice of our colleague CECCALDI and of Doctor General SALEUN, who is replacing Doctor General VAUCEL at the ministry during his holidays, Lomidinization, for reasons you know better than I, must be limited to agents who are particularly exposed due to the location of their residence or their travels. It is thus fitting that these agents ask for advice from qualified authorities who will give them all the relevant advice.

You will thus be called upon to give consultations and appropriate treatment. . . .

We can expect to see such requests grow.

You will certainly agree with us that the Instituts Pasteur must welcome them.

Noël Bernard
Director of the Institut Pasteur[60]

This was an inversion of the usual perspective: to those who wished to treat their collective staff "without any distinction," the experts responded, in the name of a rational calculation (which seems to allude to accidents), that there must be a selection of subjects for injection according to their level of risk exposure. When it came to Europeans, the risk-benefit ratio was estimated by taking into account both the real levels of exposure to the disease and the drug's risks. When it came to "the populations," however, the doctors' manuals insisted that the dangers of injection should not "lead to an underestimation of collective benefits."[61] The dividing line between individual reasoning and collective reasoning was superimposed on a line of racial distinction; in sum, one could say, an "individual" was a European.

The management of injection pain was part of this racial division. Early

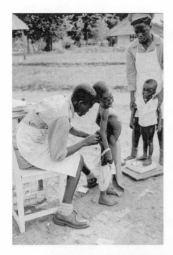
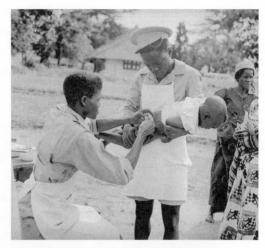
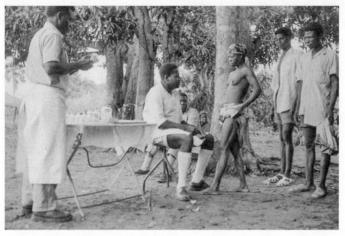

Top, pentamidinization of children in the circle of Bukanga, Kwango, Belgian Congo. "Rapport annuel du FOREAMI pour l'année 1956." © Archives of the Institute of Tropical Medicine, Antwerp. *Bottom*, Lomidine injection in Oubangui-Chari, 1956. Archives of Marinette Lugagne. All rights reserved.

studies insisted that the injections were relatively painless and did not cause complications at the site of injection. Sure, complaints were raised about the problems linked to the large volume of the doses to inject, but no systematic surveys were conducted to determine the incidence of infection, edema, or local necrosis resulting from injections. The campaigns were not suited to the follow-up of any delayed adverse events; teams were mobile by definition, and so could not monitor people for longer than a few hours after their injections. Yet the terms of this problem shifted when Lomidine was administered to a European individual. In 1949, a case of painful necrosis in a European was reported to the Institut Pasteur in Paris and warranted publication in the *Bulletin de la Société de Pathologie Exotique*.[62] A request made to Spécia is revealing of the "reality" of such pain, if such an expression can make any sense: the firm was asked to develop a combination of Lomidine with a local anesthetic, Scurocaine, because "some practitioners would like to make the injection of LOMIDINE less painful."[63] And so the pain of injection became a commercial issue, while on the ground, in African populations, this pain was ignored or mentioned only to congratulate the people on their fortitude. Yet the "shot that stings" left its mark in the oral accounts of patients and doctors: Jacques Pépin, who used pentamidine therapeutically in Zaire in the 1970s, remembers seeing men cry.[64]

To state that colonial doctors deliberately avoided evaluating the risks and benefits of pentamidinization in African patients does not imply an anachronistic judgment. Two exceptions—the British colonies and European patients —clearly reveal that this was a contingent and calculated choice, arising at the very moment when references to the racial paradigm were increasingly contested in the international arena. Pentamidine was a racialized drug. I do not mean this in the sense that its use was guided by the unescapable influence of a latent racism in doctors, but rather in the sense that its unpredictable behavior generated and rendered indispensable a racialized interpretation. The race, referring to a population conceptualized as a biological entity, was the only scale at which the drug's action and effects could be accounted for. This justified the systematic bypassing of the individual scale in evaluating both safety and efficacy. Race, as a mode of categorizing subsets of humanity, also traced the limits between individual reasoning (applied to Europeans) and collective reasoning (applied to African populations). Lomidinization was thus addressed to a strange type of being, whether an area on the map, an administrative district, or an ethnic label. To my knowledge, Lomidine, as commercialized by Spécia in 1947, is one of the only medicines to have been given an explicitly collective official indication. The leaflet specified as follows:

> Prophylaxis of trypanosomiasis (preventive Lomidinization): On the entire population of a region, administer every 4 to 6 months an injection of 3 to 4 mg of diamidino-diphenoxy-pentane per kg of body weight.[65]

Sleeping Sickness Song

Ndondo meuzeugue anga lere me nguet iben
ndondo meuzeugue anga lere me nguet ibe,
Be loum ma unlô
Be loum ma king
Be loum ma mvous
iyong bassigui aliii
Mebi me nga yi me koui
megnolok me nga yi vam
Be nga bat melom ne me keu lap mediip
Ngue me yi na ma béré assou
Man bezimbi anga sim ma ingueng unlô

(cries)
Ndondo meuzeugue anga lere me nguet iben
Ndondo meuzeugue anga lere me nguet iben.

Translation (from Hubert Ntonga's French translation)

The shot against sleeping sickness brought me so many problems
The shot against sleeping sickness hurt me so
They pricked me in the head
They pricked me in the neck
They pricked me in the back
When they go lower
Excrement wants to leave me
Urine even wants to spurt
And still, they want to send me to draw water
If I try to slow my step
The policeman hits me on the head with a stick

(cries)
The shot against sleeping sickness brought me so many problems
The shot against sleeping sickness hurt me so.

This song, in the Eton language, was sung in the 1950s in the Department of the Lékié in Cameroon. It was collected in 2005 from Hubert Mvogo, a state-qualified nurse in Yaoundé. He got it from his mother, who was from Oveng, 40 kilometers north of Yaoundé. It likely alludes to Lomidinization, which was widely used in the region. The terms used are *ndondo* (shot) and *meuzeugue* (sleeping sickness). The mention of incontinence also evokes a known effect of Lomidine. The series of "pricks" to the head, neck, and back evokes the series of punctures (in the ganglia and spine) performed for testing purposes. According to Hubert Mvogo, it was sung to "pluck up courage" during the campaigns, "because many people fled."

CHAPTER SIX

Good Citizens and Bad Brothers

> To protect yourself
> **FROM SLEEPING SICKNESS**
> To rid the country of this terrible disease for good
> **THE BEST WAY**
> is to show up unfailingly for medical screening carried out by the specialized
> health teams to receive there the injection of
> **PREVENTIVE LOMIDINE**

Insert published in the magazine *Hygiène et Alimentation au Cameroun* (*Food and Hygiene in Cameroon*), October 16, 1952, 12.

Pentamidine, that miracle solution of postwar medicine, promised to resolve the "indiscipline of recalcitrants"[1]—the term used to refer to those who avoided injection sessions. Yet this only shifted the locus of the problem. By easing the epidemic, the new drug paradoxically made the obstacle posed by indiscipline more tangible, since campaigns now aimed to eradicate the disease, that is, to achieve the ultimate contribution of colonialism to African health. Public health action needed to be kicked up a notch precisely, it might be said, because the epidemic situation had improved: "If absenteeism at preventive Lomidinization sessions could be reduced everywhere and if the sanitary control of eternal wanderers—those generous peddlers of trypanosomes—was applied everywhere in a draconian manner, the total eradication of the sleeping sickness plague could be rapidly obtained," explained Pierre Richet in 1954 to a committee of international experts gathered in Pretoria, South Africa.[2]

How could this absenteeism problem be solved? Colonial public health policies simultaneously explored two avenues that, on the surface, seemed opposed: the first was coercion through the infliction of fines and punishment, and the other was to manufacture consent through attempts to bring forth a "modern African," who would be receptive to medicine's methods and promises, including, of course, Lomidine shots. These strategies foregrounded the individual as a cause of failure and as a nuisance, but also as a transformable subject, as a potential citizen and resource for public health, who could make the eradication project his own and enroll his own kind.[3] These apparently contradictory approaches were in fact connected by a cyclical sequence of solemn declarations, generous experiments, obvious failure, and in response, ever greater ambition.

The fact that pentamidine did not work as anticipated, that it protected individuals only partially while exposing them to significant risk, did not hold these efforts back. On the contrary, the drug's misfires were fruitful on the scientific front, inspiring novel biological explanations, experiments seeking ways to prevent accidents, and a racialization of medical reasoning. The problems with pentamidine were equally productive on the political front. Being perceived merely as misunderstandings, its failures stimulated the imaginations of doctors, who designed education campaigns containing a new and surprising articulation of the issue of individual responsibility. At the same time, the drug's misses justified a series of police and military initiatives to Lomidinize, by force if necessary, individuals or villages refusing injections.

These contradictory responses were neither an accident nor a sign of "schizophrenia."[4] Confident projections and the hardening of discipline worked in tandem precisely because modern colonial medicine, no matter how generous, sought to "solve" the problems it encountered, including the problems of a drug that turned out to be more difficult to manage than expected. In this chapter I trace how the drug's misfires reinitiated colonial doctors' hyperbolic dreaming and enthusiasm.

Searching for the Modern Individual

Across Africa, postwar colonial medicine aimed to transform individuals and subjectivities, a project partly imported from the missionary medical world. The idea was to convert Africans to modernity by deploying an unprecedented educational effort.

The "hygienic education of indigenous populations" was a relatively old idea,[5] dating back to the experiments in "health propaganda" under the auspices of the Rockefeller Foundation from Europe to the Philippines just after the First World War.[6] Yet after 1945, there was a shift in its institutions, techniques, and theory. Civic and health education, a kind of hygienist evangelism, which until then had been driven by religious and philanthropic organizations, was admitted into the core vocations of the colonial state, which at the same time was adding social modernization to its objectives.

The social was thus made into a space of political intervention and imagination. A set of institutions, actors, and forms of knowledge—ranging from "psychotechnicians" (applied psychologists) and social workers to canteens and nursery schools—landed in Africa.[7] One of the distinctive characteristics of colonialism in the 1950s, as Fred Cooper has shown, was the reconstitution of an entire segment of colonial state action as a "power-knowledge regime" aimed at governing Africans. African people were no longer to be governed as "non-individualized collectivities, little known and unknowing," but instead, surely for the first time, as individuals whose assent was needed.[8] Occurring fairly late across French, Belgian, and British colonial regimes, this social (an omnipresent term in contemporary institutions) turn was part of a quest for hegemony, defined as a "peaceful extraction of consent by means of a network of institutions aiming to fashion the subjectivity of the colonized."[9] What hinged on the capacity of states to guarantee "welfare" was not only the stability of economies and homes, as was the case in Europe, but also the consent of Africans to colonial rule—and therefore the future of empires.

Colonial medicine was reorganized both in the Union française and in the Belgian Congo to address this new order. Disparate biopolitical issues and institutions, ranging from early childhood to sports, were redefined as "medico-social" as they were appropriated by the field of public health or, at least, reformulated in terms of health. This is illustrated, for instance, by the fact that the president of the Fédération camerounaise des sports (Cameroonian Sports Federation) in 1947 was none other than Raymond Beaudiment, the head of the SHMP and a great advocate of Lomidinization.[10]

More generally, imperial states developed tighter links with the missionary world, particularly with movements associated with social Catholicism. While such connections were congruous in the Belgian Congo, where missions and para-public institutions such as the FOREAMI had long been allowed to take an active role in health policies, they were more unexpected in the French case. Louis-Paul Aujoulat—a doctor, missionary, and deputy from Cameroon—embodied this convergence; from 1949 to 1953, he was one of the few Fourth Republic politicians to continuously occupy ministerial positions, including secretary of state to the Ministère de la France d'Outre-Mer and minister of health and social affairs. Linked to the congregation of the Pères du Saint-Esprit (Holy Ghost Fathers) and to a constellation of secular Catholic move-

ments, Aujoulat worked on several legislative projects pertaining to social colonial action, including the Code du travail des territoires d'outre-mer (Labor
Code of the Overseas Territories; 1952).[11] If one also considers the provision
of state support to missionary medical work and the conceptual links between
catechism and health education, one could say that the colonial government
had probably never come closer to being a "missionary administration" than
it did at that moment.[12]

Health was a strategic avenue for the transformation of subjectivity. In practice, attempts by health services to "change the African man"—attempts that
often targeted women—proliferated. In Senegal, a program of "basic education" under the auspices of the colonial government and UNESCO redesigned
the practice of hygiene lessons in schools. In the Belgian Congo, hygiene was
integrated into a set of state and missionary initiatives, notably as part of the
domestic education of young girls and women.[13] In Cameroon, several million
francs were earmarked every year for "gifts in kind to reward the assiduity
[of women in the organization Protection maternelle et infantile (Maternal
and Child Protection)]: soap, salt, meat, milk, small [items of] clothing, blan-
ket[s],"[14] with the support of the high commissioner of the republic, Robert Delavignette, who was linked to social Catholicism. Improved means of
transportation and projection made it possible to experiment with a traveling
cinema—trucks showing locally produced educational films.

Meanwhile, in the hub of colonial social sciences, the Institut français
d'Afrique noire (French Institute for Black Africa) in Dakar, researchers set up a
"'film psychology' section to study Africans' reactions to educational and rec-
reational movies."[15] In British East Africa, filmmakers concerned themselves
with audience reactions—which were usually laughter—submitting them to
scientific inquiry, complete with test screenings and expert reports.[16] Health
education became a cultural industry and an object of scientific research and
exchange. The colonial world was the field of experimentation; findings were
then imported to the metropole by social medicine figures such as Aujoulat.
The reception of educational messages, however, gave rise to countless incidents of misunderstanding: as Eric Stein has shown, colonial "theaters of
proof" were most often interpreted by colonized audiences as comedy.[17] Yet
these health education initiatives also gave rise to appropriations of corpo-
real and domestic symbols of modernity, which became markers of class for
the new African bourgeoisie. They were thus experiments in subjectification
in the Foucauldian sense of producing individuals as moral subjects who are

responsible for themselves. Finally, colonial health education was a form of popular entertainment: the beauty pageants organized by health services attracted plenty of candidates.[18]

It is important not to caricature these textual and visual productions, which stand out against doctors' usual anxieties about the out-of-control modernization of Africa. These efforts did attempt to elicit the "voice of the natives" and sought to carefully manage a real potential for appropriation. This can be better illustrated through a close look at a remarkable magazine, which was exclusively focused on health education and, from 1948, was published every trimester in Cameroon. *Hygiène et Alimentation au Cameroun* described itself as a "magazine for the African masses," with whom it "seeks to get in touch."[19] Although it was largely written by members of the SHMP, including Beaudiment, the magazine did make genuine attempts to get in touch with the African masses. "Good idea contests," "referendums," cooking recipe exchanges, letters to the editor, a "most beautiful hut contest," and the classic "baby show" sought to let the voice (and humor) of Cameroonians speak; Cameroonians, writing in French, also authored many articles.

The tables of contents of *Hygiène et Alimentation au Cameroun* can be read as an encyclopedia of modernization in action; topics included the harmful effects of alcoholism, basketball, Cameroonian cycling, the clean village, volleyball, treating minor health problems at home, and of course Lomidine. Technical messages coexisted with a broader-ranging pedagogy. Health and hygiene were associated with morality, beauty, and material prosperity. Messages were written into a linear narrative opposing backwardness to the modern individual, who "care[d] about the future of his country and of his race."[20] Individual autonomy, rather than compliance with instructions, was promoted in a way that was remarkably modern compared to contemporary educational campaigns in the metropole.[21] Articles were punctuated with slogans:

"To be clean, she uses soap."

"It is by physical education, by Sport, that the city man . . . can regain the
   strength and resistance he loses bit by bit. It is by applying Hygiene that he
   will preserve this strength and his youth better and longer than his fathers."

"The African feels a keen desire to organize his home."

"The truly modern and evolved African woman knows how to sew, and one of
   her main ambitions, quite legitimately, is to purchase a sewing machine."

"Mother . . . is the first doctor."

"Leprosy, a little perseverance can free you from it."

"Cocoa planter, the cacao tree is your best friend, all the care you give it, it will give back a hundred times in money."

"It is out of the question to treat you as little boys by prohibiting you from touching alcohol. In return, behave as men, know how to control yourselves. Use alcohol, but don't abuse it. This is the crux of the difference between the civilized [man] and the *bushman* [in English in original]. If you want to be respected, respect yourselves, don't let alcohol degrade you."[22]

Henri de Marqueissac, a veteran of the Mission Jamot who became a scientific advisor at Spécia, wrote an aphorism that graced the cover of one issue: "Submitting to medical examinations is the first step on the path of wisdom."[23]

The reception of health education campaigns is difficult to judge. These were, above all, stories that doctors told themselves, and it is tempting to just make an ironic remark and move on. Still, education worked—and not just in the eyes of the colonial administration. *Hygiène et Alimentation* printed fifteen thousand copies of each issue in 1950, and the information it carried was explicitly designed for an African public. Spécia was among its advertisers, promoting its drug Aspro (aspirin) with an image of black figures. The African individual—as responsible and as a consumer—was born. It was time to convince him to get Lomidinized.

"Injections of Health"

From Angola to Côte d'Ivoire, colonial health education sought to secure attendance at pentamidine injection sessions. For the most part, these efforts relied on simple pedagogical texts to explain the grounds for the method. Scientific truth and doctors' goodwill alone would be able to obtain trust.

In Angola, the pentamidinization brigades relied on the dissemination of tracts to convince populations that it was in their interest to receive the "injection of health"—an expression, the propaganda emphasized, coined by Africans themselves. The texts, translated into Kikongo, the language spoken in the north of Angola, did not go into details, explaining neither sleeping sickness nor pentamidine at length:

All those who have a good heart and are good negroes must contribute to this grandiose and beneficial campaign with enthusiasm and gratitude. Their help consists simply in not missing the health meetings, to not allow someone to miss them, to receive there the "injection of health."

Thus Africans, whether they are listed in the census or not, are to present themselves, by their own free will, at the fixed time and place.

Those who fail to show up are harmful not only to themselves but to everyone, spreading the disease and ruining a work in progress; they are heedless of the money and effort invested by the government. For this, they could be punished.

The authorities here content themselves with a simple logic, which they imagine to speak to the "natives": pentamidine equals future health, future fertility, and a return on the financial investments made by the colonial government, which will be in vain if there is absenteeism.

No one must miss it!!

With the help of Africans—their presence at meetings—the work of the doctors and nurses of the Health Services will be greatly facilitated and money will not be spent for nothing. This highly valuable endeavor, programmed by the Government, will bring great benefits to all in general, thanks to the increase in population that will result, and to the negroes in particular who, in the future, will not only be in better health but also have many more children.

This is why no one must be absent at the "injections of health"!!![24]

The document itself appears to have been invested with preventive powers. Portuguese doctors noted that Africans "came . . . to request a card for the 'injections of health,' which is the expression they used to refer to the bilingual (Portuguese-Kikongo) pamphlets we had printed."[25]

Some of the texts used elsewhere, for example in Cameroon, ventured a more elaborate form of scientific popularization. In 1952, *Hygiène et Alimentation au Cameroun* dedicated a long article to Lomidine, which it described as the "new drug that has been in our therapeutic arsenal for 5 or 6 years [that] allows us to boost our efforts against sleeping sickness by, as it were, vaccinating against it."[26] This article was a long effort to explain the scientific theory of Lomidinization; it particularly emphasized the importance of *total* Lomidinization, which was demonstrated, by way of numbers, in the "shining example" of the successful campaigns undertaken since 1947 in Yokadouma in the "little Bidjouki tribe." The value of Lomidinization to individuals was barely mentioned; it was assumed to be obvious. The key issue was instead the collective scale, where everyone's presence was the "primary condition" for successful protection:

The entire population, *without exception*, must receive the shot of Lomidine. It takes only a few avoiders to put the whole country in danger, since glossina[s] are so abundant along Cameroon's waterways that no one can boast of escaping their attacks. Any person who has not received the shot of Lomidine will become [infected by the trypanosome] and will create foci of contamination everywhere he goes by rendering infectious all the glossina[s] who bite him. Then it turns into a phenomenon like an oil slick or wildfire. The disease spreads from one contact to another, a threat to those who are not protected by Lomidine.

Those who refuse to receive this shot thus become a danger for the family, the village, the tribe; they behave exactly like criminals. They are bad brothers and bad Cameroonians![27]

A Political Theory of Lomidinization

The education campaigns are revealing of what they worked against: the people's apathy and antipathy. In the French colonies, absenteeism remained a major concern. Moreover, doctors worried that improvements in public health, now that new cases of sleeping sickness were becoming rarer and rarer, would further aggravate the problem. "The population might develop a sense of invulnerability that could jeopardize the rate of presence," wrote a doctor in Cameroon.[28] How paradoxical: Lomidine's success was a source of anxiety!

Allusions to the problem cropped up in doctors' correspondence: the quest for eradication made them more demanding in the face of popular avoidance and protest. In and around cities, the situation seemed particularly complicated: for example, in 1953 Jacques Pierre Ziegler wrote from Chad, in a postscript, that he had obtained "very good results on the whole, despite a very unstable and difficult population," but that he still had to tackle "the neighborhoods of Lamy [now D'Djamena], a lot of work, totally thankless and source of endless problems."[29] Police escorts were often indispensable.

This tense climate, on top of doubts about the drug's efficacy and safety, was not what unsettled doctors. Instead, in the name of the higher interest of the "race," they blamed, with increasing forcefulness, those who evaded injection during campaigns. This was not the first time, of course, that a public health campaign invoked the collective good to accuse or compel those seeking to elude medical treatment. In the United States and Europe, the hunt for germ carriers took extreme forms at times, partly as a legacy of colonial experimentation. The social prophylaxis model had political and moral implications: it designated germ carriers as threats and as pathological individuals, singling out collectives and subpopulations to be defined and treated as virus reservoirs. In the first half of the twentieth century, beginning with Typhoid

Mary, American public health's most famous "healthy carrier," the prophylaxis of infectious diseases entailed a form of political theory and practice that traced and reinforced symbolic and material barriers of race and class.[30] Epidemiology, as Paul Weindling shows with reference to European Jews, inspired the scientific racism of the 1930s and even its projects of extermination.[31] It is important to understand that the therapeutic and public health possibilities (and limits) of modern medicine *produced* racialized and repressive policies, and not that a preexisting underlying racism influenced doctors.

Pentamidinization campaigns are a good illustration of this mechanism. The method's collective interpretation was not the resurgence of an old epidemiological model. Rather, it was a novel framework created by laborious scientific efforts to give meaning to contradictions as they were encountered. Lomidinization, which doctors described as a life-size experiment, revealed by its very inability to eradicate the disease the capacity of the "floating population" to be a nuisance. Referring to "the masses" thus had a political effect. First, it obstructed the evaluation of risks and benefits at the individual scale. It also pathologized "transients and recalcitrants," identifying them scientifically as a "residual virus reservoir" that stood as the final obstacle to eradication, thus making them bear responsibility for collective failure.[32] This reasoning was untenable at the individual scale, since the stable (one might say "deserving") segment of the population was meant to be protected by their own injection no matter what proportion of the whole was actually injected. Imagined collectively, however, the failures of Lomidinization brought forth as an obstacle a group, variegated and uncertain, of pathological individuals.

"The Choice Is Yours": Lomidinization and Public Health Citizenship

Educational texts on Lomidine came up against a thorny question: How could one insist on total Lomidinization while such a demand was not directly justified by the method's principle—which was that individuals should protect themselves through their own injection regardless of others' actions? In Angola, a simple solution was devised: to appeal to hierarchy and not expect Africans to understand.[33]

In Cameroon, the contradiction inspired doctors, leading them to explore an original path in which the duty of Lomidinization would be justified in terms of membership in a community-in-the-making: the nation. A "bad brother" was also a "bad Cameroonian"; this linkage, suggested by the 1952 article cited above, was a novel one. This national reference, paradoxical at a time of emerging repression of nationalist movements, enabled a connection between the two scales of public health: the population and the individual.

An article (reproduced at the end of this chapter) entitled "A Disappearing Disease: Sleeping Sickness" dealt only briefly with the value of Lomidinization for individuals. Its first slogan, "Lomidine: Life Insurance," surely spoke more to French doctors than it did to Cameroonian readers. The discussion then moved on to collective grounds in the pursuit of a goal: "to fully wipe out sleeping sickness from Cameroon." Now the audience was Cameroonian, and the goal was for the good of Cameroon: the exhortation to Lomidinization slipped from the register of individual health to that of public health citizenship. The article's second slogan was "Are you a criminal?" Calling on the power of statistics, the danger of virus reservoirs was demonstrated. A new future burst onto the scene, a future that was no longer just the "safeguarding of the races." Now, the future of "our Cameroon" was at stake—even though this implied a highly ambiguous "us," from which the "traitors" of the UPC were excluded. This act of health propaganda concluded with an unprecedentedly civic admonition: "A village that is Lomidinized in the proportion of 100% is 100% safe from sleeping sickness. A Cameroon that is 100% Lomidinized will be a Cameroon that is rid of sleeping sickness. Cameroonians, the choice is yours."

The article's anonymous authors seem to have grasped the potential of mobilizing civic choice (it was up to "Cameroonians" to choose Cameroon's future) at a time when nationalist claims were increasingly manifest in the political sphere. In an apt slip of the pen, the article even wrote of "abstentionists" instead of absentees. By making health a civic issue, the form of health education tried in the 1950s was no longer mere medical paternalism. To borrow from Luc Berlivet's analysis, one can already perceive the outlines of a liberal form of the government of bodies, one based on imagining autonomous subjects.[34]

This unexpected invention—of propaganda for the "good citizen" who would "choose" eradication—was a last resort (recall that campaigns in Yaoundé and Douala had, at the time of the article's publication, been suspended). It was an attempt to convince the population, and perhaps also to persuade doctors themselves, that the drug still worked. This means that the propaganda was not a marginal matter: translating the logic of Lomidinization was also a method to reinforce a fragile consensus, including in the scientific arena. The message to those who were in doubt: Lomidine works; the proof is that it is being explained to the "natives" and that it is seen to carry the future of the nations to come.

It might be said, following a Latourian interpretation, that the recruitment of new allies, namely the Cameroonian people, stabilized a *fact*—the efficacy of preventive Lomidine—which was otherwise extremely tenuous. Just as population-level results had justified the elision of any assessment at the individual scale, the successful enrollment of populations, whether imagined in a text or proven by numbers, could bolster consensus about the technique. This may even have been the main function of the educational texts, which, it should be pointed out, were rather too long and complicated to have been truly instructive.

This endeavor to imagine civic adherence to Lomidine can be interpreted as a way of updating mass medicine for a new, modern Africa or, alternatively, as an attempt to prop up an edifice on the brink of collapse. Its contradictions were, it seems, a source of creativity: that the public health enterprise of a colonial state simultaneously engaged in the fierce repression of UPC nationalists could find its last fulcrum in a nationalist rhetoric of "choice" was indeed a startling paradox.

The Reactionary Option

Efforts to encourage Cameroonians to show up at injection sessions had little impact. By late 1954, the Lomidinization program had been almost completely shut down. Catastrophic accidents had made the education attempts futile. Across Africa, problems proliferated: the map of campaigns was being overlaid by a map of zones in which Lomidinization was difficult or impossible, refused en masse. Eradicating the disease was now a matter of eradicating pockets of resistance, in the literal sense of the term: epidemiological thought became openly political.

There was no shortage of reasons that any "population" might contest injection campaigns. Problematic incidents abounded, not all of which were linked to the drug itself; some also arose from medical tours' routine operations, which imposed the obligation not only to submit to medical examinations but also to supply the teams (of rarely fewer than ten people) with lodging, food, and water. The abuse of authority by nurses and health assistants had long, ever since the first sleeping sickness control campaigns, been a recurring problem (doctors, however, were almost never blamed). In Cameroon, several death penalties had been inflicted for the murder of nurses during the medical campaigns of the 1920s.[35] Usually, however, tensions were much more banal; they arose from the normal workings of colonial medicine as a form of decentralized despotism.[36] In Yokadouma, complaints were made about the African doctor: "During his tour of 13 days on [the road of the Bidjoukis] the African doctor managed to eat 15 goats, 51 kg of smoked meat and several dozen chickens. His appetite was good, but his digestion will be more difficult since the judge condemned him to a 12,000 franc fine and a suspended one-year prison sentence," wrote a missionary in 1947.[37] Meanwhile in Côte d'Ivoire, problems made their way up to the local assembly, which denounced the "raids of rice, of chickens, of kid [goats] and of silver by the agents of the SHMP, the poor treatment inflicted on recalcitrant patients and on latecomers (caning and carrying bricks)."[38] In Danané, a post that, like Yokadouma, was located on the edge of the colony, a nurse was tried in 1954 for abuse of authority.[39]

The "shot for sleeping sickness,"[40] as the missionaries called it, was also specifically feared in some areas. In retrospect, rumors of accidents seem a plausible explanation, but at the time, doctors dismissed this possibility. Rumors that the injections brought death were reported by anthropologist Tamara Giles-Vernick to be still circulating in the late 1980s in the area of Nola in Oubangui-Chari, one of the most Lomidinized in Africa.[41] In the Lékié River area in Cameroon, Lomidine is remembered with both laughter and tears: today, a song is still sung about the *ndondo meuzeugue*, a song about pain, intimidation, and beatings (see chapter 5).

The politicization of refusal was rarely explicit. Instead, it surfaced in medical reports as a threat to campaigns, especially in the two colonies where nationalist mobilization was at its most radical and best organized: in Côte d'Ivoire with the Rassemblement démocratique africain (African Democratic Assembly) and in Cameroon with the UPC. In some spots, refusal was almost unanimous; for example, in the big cities of Cameroon and Côte d'Ivoire, the low rate of presence was said to be "ridiculous."[42] This was most often merely an expression of weariness in the face of repeated campaigns. Avoiding injection was a passive gesture: all one had to do to be "absent" was to stay home. Teams usually summoned the population to points located along roads; these could be several hours' walk from people's home villages. Some died on their way back after a medical examination. For example, in Guinea a woman died in 1941 after walking 30 kilometers right after submitting to a lumbar puncture.[43]

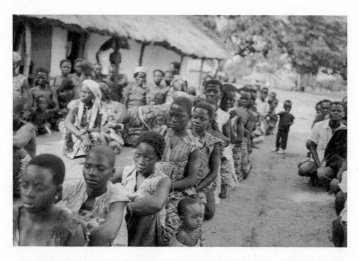

Waiting in line for pentamidinization in the circle of Bukanga, Kwango, Belgian Congo. "Rapport annuel du FOREAMI pour l'année 1956." © Archives of the Institute of Tropical Medicine, Antwerp.

These difficulties compelled doctors to innovate. The technique of checkpoints—roadblocks where travelers were intercepted and asked for proof of recent Lomidinization—was systematically applied in Côte d'Ivoire, where there was intense traffic with Guinea and Upper Volta. Maxime Lamotte, a French naturalist who worked in the Nimba Mountains region in Guinea at the time (and would, in the 1960s–70s, become a major figure of French biology), still remembered the checkpoints in the early 2000s: one day, he was required to take his place in the queue to receive the injection.[44] In Côte d'Ivoire, where people fled upon hearing that medical teams were about to arrive, the doctors resorted to a strategy of "surprise medical screenings." In Abengourou, the SGHMP showed up without warning in markets and villages to test and Lomidinize on the spot. In Gagnoa, "the doctor had to surround the village to catch the women and children who were fleeing."[45] The unpopularity of the campaigns thus grew further. By 1955, they had to be stopped.

Dr. Charles Plays War

Campaign strategists took responsibility for the escalation in the use of force. An administrator posted in Saa, Cameroon, a hotspot of Lomidinization, recounted how a young SHMP doctor organized a visit to a recalcitrant village circa 1954, a time when the disease was very nearly eradicated. His story featured someone identified only as Dr. Charles, the "chief of the Regional Service of Mobile Hygiene," who, in the region under his responsibility had come up against "spots," "enclaves" where "chiefs and populations," manipulated by UPC pro-independence fighters, "were fiercely opposed to all treatment" and refused "Lomidine, the drug that conquered the endemic."[46] The military lexicon was not just a metaphor. After poring over maps, the doctor and the administrator decided to lance the boil. They defined their strategy. Its first prong was to "motivate the chiefs," an expression still used in Cameroon in allusion to corruption: promotions and promises were handed out to local authorities. For the rest of the population, they banked on the use of force, as the region's former administrator described: "The region put at my disposal a contingent of Cameroonian guards and, at sunrise, the SHMP Base No. 33 set up in a first village, which was surrounded by the guards beforehand. The population was a little agitated, but the doctor explained, the Administrator explained, the Chief approved and recommended—for rarely do chiefs still command [these days]. Vaccination happened.[47] No one died. The UPC lied. Now we can laugh at the tsetse."[48]

This tale of victory vindicated a set of principles: the refusal of Lomidinization was a product of political manipulation, and it was a form of feminized irrationality that could be put right by way of explanations given by a doctor, who was described as "intelligent, human, competent, . . . with bottomless knowledge . . . on African health and its treatments."[49] Although the method's risks were hinted at—and indeed, fatal accidents, associated with the use of contaminated water for injections, had occurred in this very place—this was only to denounce the opportunism of independence fighters, who used this threat as a pretext to stir up agitation, "to accuse the Whites of murdering the Blacks."[50]

The political history of pentamidinization can be seen as a series of great announcements and setbacks, followed by ever more ambitious reactions. It is precisely because the drug did not work as planned that it was gradually made into a medicine for the race, to be administered without exception to all Africans in affected zones; its medical theory and political practice were founded in failure. The entire scientific history of pentamidine is thus contained in these questions, with which the doctors were obsessed: How could they make failure fit into the order of things, and how, in this way, might they redefine their mission, given its fundamental inefficacy?

That there was a contradiction between the glorious narratives of eradication-in-progress and the disorder encountered on the ground did not escape the doctors: this was their very motive for resorting to force. The failures paradox-ically strengthened doctors' determination and trust in the method. Thus, when eradication did not happen as quickly as expected, this was taken as merely (yet another) demonstration of the harmful role of recalcitrants. That a population like the Bané tribe near Yaoundé, Cameroon, "indisciplined [and] insidiously hostile to any measure taken for its own good,"[51] refused Lomidinization was simply taken as additional proof of the method's validity. Celebration of the colonial public health enterprise was thus colored by the disappointment felt by the doctors themselves: that its success was incomplete and misunderstood only confirmed the greatness and selflessness of their mis-sion. Doctors were already, in the postwar years, catching a whiff of the end of empire.

> A few small spots on the map will still remain, which I will not have time to erase; I will leave these to my successor.
>
> Doctor Charles! How many thousand Africans owe you their lives? How many of their descendants are aware of this? Are they grateful to you? The Doctor does not think so. He has been around and has lost his illusions. Like me, he loves his work. And he will do it well, whether or not his patients love him for it.[52]

Generous fictions of social colonialism, calls for a return to order, reaction, and melancholy: the literary production of colonial medicine kept moving from one register to another. Public health was thus located simultaneously at the vanguard both of the colonial emancipatory imagination and of co-lonial repression. The relationship between the epidemiology of eradication and police operations was a two-way street: from 1958, the French army ex-perimented with "psychological action" in Cameroon to supplement acts of "pacification" in its attempt to destabilize the UPC's underground networks in Bassa country. Medical propaganda provided a fulcrum. A simple slogan, devised by military experts who would later carry their ideas into the Algerian conflict, was whitewashed onto walls in the area: "UPC = tsetse; it bites, it puts to sleep, it kills."[53]

A Disappearing Disease
SLEEPING SICKNESS

There are many who remember! That time was barely twenty-five years ago. Sleeping sickness wreaked such havoc that vast regions were at risk of disappearing from the ethnological map and becoming vast hunting reserves haunted only by wild animals. . . .

A new drug, for which scientists from many countries had worked hidden away in their laboratories, was then implemented against sleeping sickness. . . .

LOMIDINE: LIFE INSURANCE

Lomidine is real life insurance against sleeping sickness.

In addition to the immediate, selfish, personal benefits that each Cameroonian can expect from being Lomidinized, there is another reason that must urgently compel each Cameroonian to accept the shot of Lomidine, this reason is that Lomidine can make sleeping sickness disappear completely from Cameroon, as long as the totality of the population of contaminated zones gets preventively Lomidinized.

Lomidine can make sleeping sickness disappear just like . . . vaccination made yellow fever disappear from all the countries of [sub-Saharan] Africa. Unfortunately, because of the indiscipline of populations of our Cameroon, we are still far from realizing this beautiful dream of total Lomidinization.

Yet there is a means of protecting oneself from the ever-present danger of being bitten by an infected fly and becoming both ill and a virus reservoir: it is to get the shot of Lomidine twice a year. Lomidine stays in the blood for about six months and if, during this time, a tsetse bites you and inoculates you with trypanosomes, these microbes, on contact with the Lomidine in the blood, will die within a few hours. By getting Lomidinized, not only will you no longer be exposed to this affliction, but also—and this is important for the future of Cameroon—you will no longer be at risk of becoming a virus reservoir that can spread the disease.

ARE YOU A CRIMINAL?

You can see how the person who avoids Lomidinization sessions behaves exactly like a criminal.

If the totality of the population of a village that was summoned to Lomidinization showed up for the shot, it could be mathematically asserted that this village will never get sleeping sickness. But if ten or twenty persons out of a hundred hide and flee from the shot, we can say that, mathematically, there is a ten to twenty percent chance that someday this village will be contaminated. These abstentionists are thus a danger for the rest of the village, and it is not an exaggeration to say that they behave like criminals toward their brothers. It is up to the chiefs of the groupings, who guide the opinion of the natives, to grasp the significance of these facts, and to explain to those around them so that all their villagers go to Lomidinization. . . .

To sum up, we can assert that with today's drugs, and especially with that wonderful drug Lomidine, we are sure of eliminating sleeping sickness from Cameroon in fewer than five years, if you help us by coming, all of you, to vaccination sessions.

A village that is Lomidinized in the proportion of 100% is 100% safe from sleeping sickness. A Cameroon that is 100% Lomidinized will be a Cameroon that is rid of sleeping sickness. Cameroonians, the choice is yours.

Hygiène et Alimentation au Cameroun 19 (July 1, 1953), 6–7, 14.

CHAPTER SEVEN

Yokadouma, Cameroon, November–December 1954

REPORT THAT FOLLOWING LOMIDINE VACCINATION 5 DEATHS AND SEV-
ERAL SERIOUSLY ILL—STOP—HAVE TELEGRAPHED CAPTAIN-DOCTOR CON-
STANT TO COME VERY URGENTLY—STOP—PLEASE VERY URGENTLY INITIATE
PUBLIC HEALTH INQUIRY [signed] GILBRIN[1]

On the morning of Monday, November 15, 1954, a telegram (quoted above) arrived at the Direction de la santé publique (Public Health Directorate) in Yaoundé; it was sent by Gilbrin (his full name is unknown), the chief regional officer of the region of Boumba-Ngoko, from its capital, Yokadouma. It carried news of five deaths following injections of Lomidine. Later that morning, the postal clerk of Yokadouma transmitted more telegrams: one called in Captain Yves Constant, the doctor in chief of the neighboring region of Lom and Kadei, as reinforcement; another alerted the High Commission, the seat of the French administration in Cameroon. Officials in Yaoundé were being made aware of a catastrophe unfolding more than 500 kilometers east of the capital, near the border with Oubangui-Chari (AEF). At the dispensary in Yokadouma, the toll of the catastrophe grew by the hour.

These events in Yokadouma mark a turn in Lomidine's history. Until late 1954, incidents arising in the course of campaigns reinforced, rather than destabilized, the core set of knowledge, beliefs, and practices underlying mass interventions. The catastrophic events narrated in this chapter, however, raised questions, at least briefly, about the method's trustworthiness. The Yokadouma catastrophe can be called a "test," following Luc Boltanski's use of the term: an exceptional moment in which the order of the world—here, the social, racial, moral, and epistemological hierarchies that defined, far beyond the issue of the drug's safety, colonialism itself—was questioned, disturbed, and ultimately, rearranged.[2]

"The Tour Was Proceeding as Usual"

The region of Yokadouma was a hotspot of Lomidinization, often cited as a case example in propaganda articles. In 1948, at a time of dramatic resurgence in the incidence of sleeping sickness, it was the site of the first trials in Cameroon. The rubber boom of the Second World War had aggravated the region's ecological volatility, fanning an epidemic flare-up on both sides of the border. Whether compelled by the administration or attracted by a hike in prices, local peasants had rushed into the forest to collect as much latex as they could, exposing themselves to tsetse flies.

Applied to the entire region, Lomidinization made it possible to bring the epidemic under control: as early as 1949, only a handful of new cases were detected, and the incidence rate was near zero. Yet for doctors, the disease remained a threat, especially when in 1950 "six Europeans" were infected in Yokadouma itself.[3] Thus, Lomidinization continued, repeated once or twice a year on almost the whole population registered in the census. In 1954, more than sixteen thousand individuals were examined, and no new cases were found.[4] Across the border in the region of Nola, which was contiguous with AEF, chemoprophylaxis was applied with the same zeal and success: the prevalence rate dropped from 24 percent in 1943 (a quarter of the population infected) to zero in 1952.[5]

In November 1954, the SHMP's Groupe mobile de traitement (GMT; Mobile Treatment Group) number 15 set off to Lomidinize the cantons of Yangéré and Mbimou, situated along the road to the city of Batouri. The team had no doctor; it was headed by a contracted, locally recruited European "health assistant," M. Ansellem, who had "four African nurses" under his supervision.[6]

The team left from its base in Batouri on the morning of November 5. According to protocol, Ansellem began with a visit to the chief regional officer in Yokadouma, to initiate arrangements with local chiefs for the gathering of the population. The following day, still in Yokadouma, around fifty people showed up at the dispensary to receive their shot of Lomidine. This number is indicative of the small size of the regional capital, which was a mere administrative outpost at the heart of one of the most remote and sparsely populated regions of Cameroon. For the men posted out there, it represented an "end of the world," a "place to stick loony administrators,"[7] wrote a missionary at the time, while a doctor described it as a "scattering of tiny villages."[8]

On the morning of November 7, the campaign officially began 60 kilometers north of the city. The plan was to advance, day by day, back toward Yokadouma, summoning the population to meeting points along the road, which were designated by their distance markers (for example, at "kilometer 17"). Up until the evening of November 10, more than five hundred injections were administered each day. The presence rate was high—the region did not have a reputation for being "difficult"—and the local chiefs were cooperative. The team then took a day off so that Ansellem could call on the manager of the neighboring Kulikowski plantation.

The medical team's work resumed on November 12 at the meeting site of Gribi, 30 kilometers from Yokadouma. Lomidine solution was, as usual, prepared on the spot by mixing Spécia powder into a solution, using water that had been filtered and then sterilized by boiling. More than 500 individuals gathered, lined up, and were injected in the buttocks. The next day, another 650 individuals showed up in Gribi and were Lomidinized in a few hours. Ansellem then left Gribi to spend the night in Yokadouma, "when suddenly the following events occurred."[9]

Excerpt from the report of Chief Regional Officer Gilbrin

French Republic

Liberté—Égalité—Fraternité

Territory of Cameroon—Region of the Boumba-Ngoka [*sic*]

No. 142 CF/RBN

ANALYSIS

Fatal accidents following passage [of] GMT 15

[stamped] CONFIDENTIAL

Yokadouma, November 19, 1954

CHIEF OF REGION OF THE BOUMBA-NGOKO

HIS EXCELLENCY THE HIGH COMMISSIONER OF THE FRENCH REPUBLIC IN CAMEROON (GENERAL SECRETARIAT)—YAOUNDÉ

I have the honor of reporting that a series of fatalities has just occurred in the region of the Boumba-Ngoko, following Lomidinization treatment by the GMT 15, in two cantons of the region.

A Mobile Treatment Group (GMT 15) under the supervision of M. ANSELLEM, health assistant of the SHMP, assisted by four nurses, vaccinates [*sic*] for trypanosomiasis the whole population of the subdivision of YOKADOUMA, with shots of the Lomidine solution every semester. No accident had yet occurred during this vaccination.

The GMT 15 had planned a Lomidinization program covering the cantons of Yangéré and Mbimou from the 8th to the 16th of this month. These two cantons are situated on the track that leads from YOKADOUMA to BATOURI.

The population was notified by the local administration that they had to show up for these vaccination sessions, which take place at each center of a cluster of villages.

This public health tour was proceeding as usual when suddenly the following events occurred (I list them chronologically):

Saturday 11/13, 8 p.m. A truck from the KULIKOWSKI plantation (situated 50 km from YOKADOUMA) brings to YOKADOUMA a patient presenting with a large swelling at the site of injection. The patient is driven to the dispensary.
The truck's driver mentions, without giving much detail, that there are other cases.

Sunday, 14, noon M. ANSELLEM, who had returned to Yokadouma on Saturday evening, goes back to the GMT 15's site of operation, to continue his public health tour and to check on the patients that were declared.
5 p.m.: The African doctor BOTETEME, supervisor of the health post of YOKADOUMA, tells me that the patient brought the previous evening is better.
5:30 p.m.: M. ANSELLEM is back in YOKADOUMA and informs me of three deaths and a number of cases of illness among those recently vaccinated.
6 p.m.: The KULIKOWSKI plantation truck brings to YOKADOUMA 21 people who appear to be more or less gravely ill, all had been vaccinated—Are hospitalized at once.
I immediately write an [official telegram], top priority to request that the regional doctor in chief, based in BATOURI, come immediately—Because of radio working hours, this [official telegram] can only be sent on Monday the 17th [sic] at 7 a.m.
6–8 p.m.: The African doctor BOTETEME assisted by his nurses hospitalize and begin to treat 21 patients.
8:15 p.m.: The African doctor BOTETEME makes his way by pickup [truck] to these patients' villages to check out the public health situation, and see what he can treat.
Separation of the nurses of YOKADOUMA into two groups:

First group accompanies the African doctor BOTETEME—
Second group for the treatment of the patients who have just arrived.

I give the order to M. ANSELLEM to cease all Lomidinization operations immediately, to stay in YOKADOUMA with his nurses of the GMT 15.

<u>Monday, 11/15, 7:30 a.m.</u> Situation at the YOKADOUMA dispensary:

Two fatalities during the night
Four or five patients are in a coma

Six new patients were brought to the dispensary during the night (all from the same villages).
The serious cases have symptoms of gas gangrene (swelling—putrefaction of the tissues —bursting) at the site of the injection—(sometimes, but rarely, elsewhere, the face for example).
I send M. HANSKERS [deputy regional officer] on the road to take stock of the situation and to bring back the serious cases, by truck, to YOKADOUMA, as well as the African doctor BOTETEME.
I stay in YOKADOUMA to provide reassurance—huge crowds at the dispensary where the families of the deceased, of patients, villagers flock from all sides. Under these circumstances, I do not want to suddenly deploy the police, so I remain on the alert all morning to keep any agitation in check.
8:30 a.m: I retelegraph captain-doctor CONSTANT to describe the situation and order him to come immediately to YOKADOUMA.
Reports issued by [official telegrams] to

Secretary-General
Director of Health
Head of the S.H.M.P.

I apologize for not being able to send these [official telegrams] in code, for lack of time, for the reasons laid out above, being alone here.
9:30 a.m.: Another death
10:30 a.m.: Another death
2:15 p.m.: Arrival in YOKADOUMA of Captain-Doctor CONSTANT—not long before the return of Mr. HANSKERS and the African doctor BOTETEME.[10]

Dr. Théodore Botétémé, the "African doctor"[11] in charge of Yokadouma's dispensary (which means that, under normal circumstances, he was the only doctor in the region), updated Dr. Constant, who had just arrived from Batouri to help out. All affected villages were located near Gribi. Nearly three hundred people had been identified as suffering—the diagnosis was now supported by evidence—from gas gangrene.

Care was arranged. Constant, who had brought medicines, began to treat patients, who were triaged according to their state, at the dispensary. He gave sulfonamides to all patients; in the most serious cases, he lanced abscesses, cleaned the wounds, and tried to keep patients alive with cardiac stimulants, gas gangrene antitoxin, and penicillin; there wasn't enough of these medicines for everyone. Nurses were sent to the villages to organize on-site treatment centers in order to avoid transporting patients to Yokadouma, which might jeopardize both their health and "public order."[12]

The afternoon was tense. "The population has crowded in front of the dispensary—dispersion is delicate and difficult."[13] Ansellem shut himself off at home; the crowd was threatening him and his nurses. A form of "mob justice" was zeroing in on the chief of the mobile team.[14] His hut was attacked. "Threats—screams—rocks thrown," one official report would put it.[15] A tree was felled across the road to stop the team from going anywhere.[16] The chief regional officer, with the help of the canton chiefs and Dr. Constant, calmed the unrest without resorting to force; until further notice, Ansellem was to be kept in custody in his office, guarded by three Cameroonian police auxiliaries. With the available trucks, Gilbrin arranged to have bodies and grieving families returned to their home villages.

On November 16, the list of casualties grew longer. Around forty cases of severe gangrene were under treatment. By the evening, when Colonel-Doctor Cauvin (first name unknown), the head of the SHMP, bearing stocks of gas gangrene antitoxin, arrived from Yaoundé to begin the medical investigation, the death toll had reached twenty-four. The following day, he was joined by other authorities: the justice of the peace and the chief of police arrived from Batouri to open a judicial inquiry; a man identified only as Christol, the inspector of administrative affairs, representing the high commissioner, arrived from Yaoundé on a "special airplane";[17] he was accompanied by René Mindjos, the elected representative of the region to the Territorial Assembly, the ATCAM (under the 1946 Constitution of the Union française, the French colonies were given elected parliaments).

The following days were calmer. The antibiotic treatment was effective, and by November 18 the health situation was stabilizing; although a few patients were still in critical condition, no new serious cases were reported. On that evening, six days after the accident, a "rescue mission," composed of a doctor, a pharmacist, and nurses, arrived from Yaoundé by truck with supplies of penicillin. Together, the chief regional officer, Counselor Mindjos, and Inspector Christol visited the "bush treatment centers" set up in affected villages, promising compensation to the victims' families.[18] On November 19, they sent a reassuring telegram to the high commissioner: "The patients are treated by 10 African nurses, the auxiliary doctor, the doctors of medicine Constant and Cauvin. . . . No new death is to be deplored and no complications are to be feared other than scars on the leg wounds."[19]

The worst was over. The time for reports had come: the chief regional officer sent in his report, giving an hour-by-hour account of events, while the inspector of administrative affairs and the director of the SHMP returned to the territorial capital to write theirs. The judicial inquiry, "an investigation of X [person or persons unknown] for involuntary manslaughter,"[20] continued as the section's police chief, the attorney general, and the chief justice arrived from Yaoundé. Over the following week, the coming and going of officials dwindled, and peace returned to the post, despite two further fatalities during the night of November 24. The most critically ill were finally evacuated, first to Batouri on November 30, and then by airplane to Yaoundé for surgery. At the end of the month, the official toll was 28 deaths, 17 cases that had been "critical," another 117 that were "serious," 70 that were "less serious," and 113 that experienced "slight reactions."[21]

Ordering the Catastrophe

I was able to write the account above on the basis of reports produced immediately after these events. Narration, with its rhythms and its effects, is a bureaucratic technique, a tool of imperial government that my own text could not circumvent.[22] Although archived, these reports were not written for historians: beyond the facts described, the act of reporting itself has a logic and a political role, which must also be taken into account. To set events into an account is also to set them in order.

The reports were submitted within the span of fewer than ten days. First to arrive were the reports of the chief regional officer, Gilbrin, which were sent to the High Commission five days after the first case was detected, and then in succession arrived the reports of the inspector of administrative affairs, Christol; Lieutenant-Colonel Cauvin, the head of the SHMP; and finally, the chief of police on November 26.[23] At the end of the month, the monthly political report of the chief regional officer joined the stack of typed pages at the Directorate of Political and Administrative Affairs of the High Commission in Yaoundé.[24] All these reports had two explicit objectives in common: to give an account of the administration's mobilization in response to the catastrophe and to shed light on the causes of the deaths. Yet beyond these immediate tasks, the reports also participated in a broader enterprise: to make sense not just of an accident, but of a crisis that shook the colonial order, and moreover, to resolve this crisis by fitting these events into the logics and categories of colonial government.

The reports' authors first described the mobilization of their fellow officers. They began with detailed chronologies, accurate to the quarter of an hour, of the Lomidinization campaign and continued with descriptions of the situation as it unfolded. These official narratives, punctuated by dates and hours, portrayed the intervention of agents of the state—toward the crowd, for example—as decisive and dramatic. The story thus recreated an atmosphere of urgency, conjured by the pile of telegrams attached to the files; incidentally, it also provided an explanation for the haste of officials. It made colonial figures into men of action, overshadowing other characters. The African doctor Théodore Botétémé, although he was present from the very beginning and was congratulated after the events, vanished from the narrative as soon as French doctors arrived in Yokadouma on the afternoon of November 15. Nurses and local chiefs hardly appeared at all. The colonial state's representatives, featured at the heart of the action by the very form of the reports, then turned themselves into detectives and sociologists.

The major portion of the reports dealt with the question of what caused the fatalities. The inquiry had begun as soon as the head of the SHMP arrived in Yokadouma on November 16. Dr. Cauvin undertook the task of collecting the individual index cards associated with each of the deceased during the Lomidinization process. A few bodies were even exhumed to retrieve cards buried with them. The Lomidine powder was seized, the discarded ampules were tracked down at the gathering sites, and the water used for the solution was collected. Cauvin and some subsequent investigators also interviewed the nurses, Ansellem, and a few villagers for detailed accounts of the campaign. A reconstruction was even planned. By November 17, samples of both water and Lomidine were taken to Yaoundé and Douala for analysis. Finally, on the basis of data provided by Constant, clinical information was collected for all cases.

Positing a diagnosis was not difficult. Indeed, it had been immediately clear at the site of the incidents; the symptoms were quite obvious. The diagnosis was gas gangrene, a problem familiar to military doctors, who were conversant with its clinical description, treatment protocols, and etiology. This deadly infection was known to be caused by *Bacillus perfringens* (the term used by

French doctors; in English, the name *Clostridium welchii* was commonly used), a bacteria that is found in outside environments in the form of encysted and highly resistant spores that grow well in tissues damaged by war wounds or medical procedures; they release gas and deadly toxins.[25] Rather, the challenge was to make the accident tellable by fitting it into a chain of causal relations and to make a show of the investigators' deductive method and impartiality.

Without waiting for the analytical results, the head of the SHMP launched into an epidemiological exercise as part of his report. His reasoning, which would later be restated by other officials, was based on rather simple deductions. Analysis of the cards first revealed that all the deceased had been Lomidinized on November 12 at the gathering site at Gribi. A few cases of less serious complications had been Lomidinized on the thirteenth. The Lomidine used on November 12 was from the same batch as the powder used on other days between November 9 and 14. There was also no change in the method of preparation and injection, which complied with official recommendations. By means of a summary table, Cauvin demonstrated that only one factor had varied: the water used to prepare the solution and, more specifically, the filter used to purify it. On the twelfth, and only on that day, water had been drawn from the home of the Kulikowski plantation's manager and treated by the nurses using the plantation's filter while, on the other days, the water, drawn from various wells, was filtered with the team's Esser filter.[26] The Lomidine itself, Cauvin concluded, was thus "exonerated," and there was "incontestably" an "infectious factor present," as confirmed by the "symptomatology and [the] remarkable efficacy of treatment with antibiotics and gas gangrene antitoxin."[27]

Where did the germs come from? Probably not from tainted syringes, needles, or Lomidine ampules, for the ampules had been properly sealed, and it was unlikely, given the number of infections, that the syringes and needles were repeatedly contaminated. The remaining variable was the water in the solution, of which several cubic centimeters were injected into each patient. The scenario of the accident followed: "The water taken from the plantation is the only suspect and must have contained spores"; the "spores, not destroyed by sterilization, found a highly favorable environment in tissues made ischemic by injected Lomidine."[28] The presence of spores in the water was surely due to a defect in the plantation's filter, if we can believe "Mister Ansellem's boy," who drew the water and "assert[ed] having taken it into the filter." Cauvin concluded: "It is the only logical explanation we can give these accidents. The product and staff are not to be held responsible because . . . we cannot blame the team's chief for not having personally filled the bottles with filtered water. The team chief cannot do everything himself."

Neither the product, the material, the methods, nor the staff were responsible; that was the conclusion drawn by Dr. Cauvin, which would be taken up by the rest of the administration. The deaths were caused by invisible defects in a filter and the presence of spores. The laboratory analyses underway were expected to confirm the presence of spores in the filtered water and in the victims; the quintessential Pasteurian act would uncover the gas gangrene germ.

A Colonial Theory of Knowledge

Placed alongside the diligence of the investigators, the popular interpretations and reactions appeared to be incoherent. The epistemology of colonialism relies on what Ann Stoler calls "hierarchies of credibility";[29] these were both mobilized and confirmed by the administrators' documentary labors. Although the head of the SHMP did try to ask villagers about the physical sensations caused by Lomidine injections, "the residents [we] questioned gave different answers from one village to another, and sometimes even from one village neighborhood to another. . . . For some the shot was clearly more painful, for others there was no difference with shots received earlier, and for a few others, the shot was less painful than usual."[30] And if, "on the whole, it seems to emerge from the large number of interviews that the[se] injections were more painful than [those of] previous Lomidinization sessions," it was difficult to make use of these "more or less biased" responses. "Some," added the SHMP director, "go as far as to actually claim they suffered temporary blindness that healed completely!" He was surprised by this reemergence of a "memory of accidents caused by tryparsamide 20 or 25 years ago."

The African nurses were hardly more reliable for the purposes of the investigation. The possibility of sabotage was not ruled out, and the nurses were prime suspects; at the SHMP, nurses were accused on a regular basis of lacking "moral standards." "It is not impossible," suggested Inspector Christol, "[indeed] this has happened before—that the nurses intentionally contaminated a syringe or a medicine to make trouble for their supervisors or for villagers."[31] He then added, shrewdly: "The idea of contaminating the water would occur to someone who did not want to be accused of having given a shot with a dirty syringe or needle."[32] The accusations made by the people and their violent reactions targeting the team's supervisor reinforced such suspicions and created an opening for detailed descriptions of the frictions that normally surrounded mobile health interventions:

> [The villagers] ask for the health assistant to be punished, who in their eyes is guilty at least of negligence or incompetence or of malice. For a while, the villagers have been complaining a little that Mr. Ansellem and the nurses have been ordering more supplies than the ration. . . . Apparently, there was also quarreling between the nurses and the villagers about women and an African merchant thinks that the nurses put a bad medicine in the shots to get revenge on the villagers, without the knowledge of the health assistant.[33]

None of these accusations were really taken seriously, especially given that the defective filter scenario did not need anyone to be found guilty of the accident; the police report even "excluded" the hypothesis of malicious intent.[34] Yet by giving detailed accounts of what the people had said, the expertise of investigators could move from an analysis of the accident to the analysis of a problem that was no less preoccupying for the colonial state: popular reactions.

The reports went beyond merely mentioning the "mob justice" that shook up Yokadouma following the first fatality. They gave meticulous descriptions of its manifestations and of the "sangfroid" with which agents of the state managed the situation.[35] They praised the "reflexes" of the chief regional officer, in particular his "insight into African reactions," which had given him the ability to calm the population.[36] In the inspector's report, the villagers' overly emotional response, unfolding in "three phases," was interpreted in psychological terms:

a. Their first feeling was one of profound emotion that turned into hostility, clearly directed against the health assistant. This collective explosion of rage was rapidly dispelled due to the intervention of Mr. Gilbrin [the chief regional officer].

b. Then worry and sadness took over everyone who had been injected. They wondered whether they were all going to die or go blind. The improvement seen in patients following the care given by Dr. Constant and his aides, the ceasing of the deaths, the solicitude of the administration gradually brought back a feeling of trust.

c. Finally, we are starting to see genuine optimism at the prospect of a forthcoming payment of administrative compensation.[37]

Highly emotional and full of imagination, the people rescued by the administration were also self-interested. Investigators all considered compensation to be the main guarantee of appeasement, but only as long as it happened quickly: here, again, it was necessary to manage the population's unpredictability. "Already rumors [about the amounts promised] are circulating," warned the chief regional officer.[38] These amounts were at risk of becoming, "in villagers' imagination, sums out of proportion with what they would normally be allocated."[39]

The people were even suspected of fraud: two long pages of the medical report were filled with a detailed study of three cases of death that villagers had imputed to Lomidinization—no doubt because of the compensation being announced—but that Dr. Cauvin refused to include as casualties of the accident. In all three cases, the Lomidinization cards had disappeared, and the witness testimonies were contradictory. Two of the corpses were dug up for the investigation: one was an "old alcoholic" man, the other was a woman. In the absence of an injection scar, neither of the deaths could be attributed to Lomidinization, concluded Cauvin; thus he exposed two cheats and lightened an already heavy death toll.

On one side: incoherence, emotionality, venality; on the other: action, science, justice. The medical anthropology of the colonial authorities drew on its classics by studying "the state of mind of the population."[40] The conclusions of their expert assessments sanctioned the normal order of colonial values—a racialized distribution of reliability, morality, reason, and emotion. Calm had returned, and "the villagers have not lost their trust in the Health Services." Even better, "they also ask that a European doctor be permanently posted in Yokadouma."[41] For locals, this was a way of complaining about the marginal status of the region, where the only health personnel were two subalterns, an African doctor, and a health assistant; for the French, it was an assertion of the value of colonial medicine.

Even the reports' most significant recommendation—to suspend all campaigns in the region—paradoxically reinforced the usual assumptions. This measure did not entail a reevaluation of the method's risks, but rather sought to take into account the irrational reactions of people who would now surely flee at sight of the drug. To resume the campaigns would be "a political mistake and a demographic disaster," warned the chief regional officer.[42] For the same reasons, Ansellem would have to be removed from the region regardless of the eventual conclusions of the judicial inquiry: in Cameroon "his name [would] now be associated in the mind[s] of African villagers with the deaths caused by Lomidinization."[43]

The head of the SHMP did not question the suspension of campaigns; he even went as far as suggesting the need to restrict Lomidinization to "very limited areas" in the future. Still, he worried about this and reaffirmed his trust in Lomidinization: "At this time, systematic Lomidinization has been stopped across the whole territory, but this can only be a temporary solution if we want to prevent a resurgence of trypanosomiasis."[44] The inspector of administrative affairs envisioned the future in similar terms, that is, irrational populations, an infallible technique, and a pragmatic administration. He suggested "hold[ing] out until the population itself, aware of an eventual reemergence of trypanosomiasis, demands, insistently, the resumption of preventive Lomidinization."[45]

The World Back on Its Feet

To conclude this discussion of the documents produced immediately after the catastrophe of Yokadouma, I could paraphrase one of their own conclusions: by the end of November 1954, "this sorry affair [had] ended in terms of protecting public order."[46] However, the order that had been restored was not just the "public order." It referred also to a more general arrangement, a set of social and racial hierarchies and a way of ordering knowledge and ignorance and also reason and emotion within society. More specifically, it was the epistemology—in the sense of a theory of knowledge—of colonial power that had been protected, including the definition of what constituted reliable testimony or proof, the uneven distribution of knowledge and rationality across society, and the relations of domination and trust that this distribution implied.

This order had been destabilized during the few hours when corpses were piling up at the hospital of Yokadouma, when the telegraph was unavailable, when Constant was spending an ordinary Sunday in Batouri, when Yaoundé knew nothing of the incident, when Ansellem was being accused and attacked, and when Lomidine, having brought death, was dangerous. The crisis had been real, but now order was back; everyone had again found their place, their role, and their attributes. The population proved emotional yet faithful: "It gives itself over to the diligence of the administration and of the judicial service to obtain reparation."[47] Similarly, "the African doctor and his staff acted with devotion,"[48] while Constant, a young colonial doctor, "by his

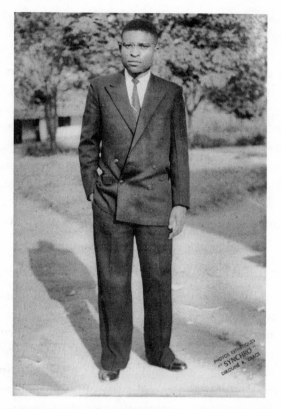

Théodore Botétémé, circa 1953. Botétémé family archives. All rights reserved.

quick action, the soundness of his diagnosis and of treatment, certainly saved many lives." The justice of the peace acted with "understanding" and "seriousness," the postal clerk with "competence," the manager of the plantation with "devotion" by lending his truck. The counselor to the assembly, Mindjos, "refrained from any offensive or acerbic comment," the dug-up corpses were reburied, and the "sick Christian women of the villages were able to receive the succor of religion by the care of the Cameroonian abbot before they died." Neither the principle nor the methods of Lomidinization were in question; it was simply a matter, in the future, of "giving the team chiefs the means of achieving perfect asepsis." The process of reassurance was complete: "The population trusts in the administration and in justice"; "it was very touched by the gesture of the High Commissioner . . . and has asked [that he] be thanked."

One might even say, following Bruno Latour, that the intervention of "nonhuman actors"—the spores, the filter, penicillin—is what allowed order to return, that establishing order in the natural world corresponds to the reestablishment of social order.[49] The epidemiological treasure hunt and a crack in a water filter did not just exonerate Lomidine, explain the crisis, and enlighten high officials; penicillin, sulfonamides, and gas gangrene antitoxin did not just save a few patients. They righted, for a moment, the colonial society as it had worked in Boumba-Ngoko when the GMT 15 set out in early November 1954 to start its latest Lomidinization campaign.

C'est fort la France!

Paule Constant was ten years old in November 1954 when her father received a telegram calling him to come at once, with medicines and materials, to Yokadouma. The "epidemic of gas gangrene" is part of her family history, a story that may not have been told to the children but was retold around the adults' table. Paule Constant has since written a dozen novels. She was awarded the Goncourt Prize in 1998.

This Lomidinization accident is the focus of her novel published in 2013, *C'est fort la France!* (*France Is Awesome!*). The book features the colonial society of Batouri confronting the shock of an accident arising during a sleeping sickness eradication campaign. I discovered the novel by chance in a bookstore, attracted by its dust cover: a pretty picture of Paule Constant as a child on the veranda of a colonial bungalow. This was the residence of Batouri's doctor in chief, who, at the time, was her father, Yves Constant, born in 1919 in Oran and posted in Cameroon after serving in the Indochina War. The novel is fictionalized yet based on history: the team's chief, a "petit Blanc" (low-ranking European), is named Bodin; the gangrene was caused by a medicine called "Lomidon," which was dissolved in poorly filtered water; the accident happened somewhere in the forest, far from Batouri, among a tribe, the Sennous (in French, a wordplay on *c'est nous*, meaning "that's us"). The residents of two villages assembled, two hundred were injected, about a hundred fell ill, and a dozen died. An angry crowd formed a barricade and killed a nurse; a string of officials passed through Batouri's airport to fly to the site; a young doctor, Constant, provided emergency care, was congratulated, then forgotten, and became annoyed at "an incompetent administration that knows nothing about anything it commands."[50] Before I caught on to who Paule Constant is, I thought a novelist had plagiarized my thesis!

There is little a historian can do with this text, which cannot be used as a source and yet cannot be ignored. Constant's words recreate, perhaps better than mine can, the turning of a world upside down: "Nothing had remained in its place, anything could happen."[51] Her words evoke the terror that must have seized the doctors Botétémé and Constant as they stood at night in the Yokadouma dispensary, powerless in the face of agony. Her words tell of gangrene and moaning, of surgery without morphine, of not enough penicillin, of the "disease of dead and rotten legs,"[52] of the pit in which amputated legs were thrown, of the nameless dead. But words can never truly capture the carnage.

CHAPTER EIGHT

"We Cried without Making a Palaver"

Of course, in the end it was a heavy blow because people died. . . . Because there was a scandal. It ended in scandal. . . . It was before . . . we were in Ayos [in 1958]. We don't know how that Lomidine was prepared. People died.

It created a big scandal?

It created a big scandal but because there was a lot more good than bad, they said it's an accident and that's how it was dealt with.

And people complained?

Heh . . . "people complained." It was back in the day. . . . Where would they go to complain?

—Interview with Samuel Menga (senior laboratory technician, retired, Pasteur Center of Cameroon, and former nurse, Public Health Service, 1958–60), Yaoundé, 2005.

The administration's mobilization following the accident at Yokadouma was a security operation, a show of strength; the aim was to maintain public order. Yet the investigators were uneasy; their actions and sweaty palms were those of a nervous colonial state. The authorities were aware of the limits of their expertise: there were gray areas their sociology was unable to grasp, anger and fear in these men despite their "sangfroid," doubts about the drug's value and safety. The administrative inspector's report thus ended by pointing out a peculiar phenomenon: "The African clerks are of the opinion that the drug is bad. . . . [They] are very reluctant to be Lomidinized."[1] But there was no need to get too worried, since "there is no notorious agitator in Yokadouma." Still, Inspector Christol added, "it is not impossible that some might go there to give their version of events."[2] A shadow was cast. In fact, this shadow had haunted Yokadouma ever since the catastrophe began: the menace, marginal and anecdotal yet palpable, of a "few fanatics," "agitators," and "opponents," the danger of "politics" and "palaver."[3] For a brief moment of uncertainty over a few days in mid-November, this shadow threatened to make a scandal, even an affair of state, of the accident. Lomidine became a matter of concern in Yaoundé and beyond—in Paris, Brussels, and Vitry-sur-Seine—while accusations and rumors proliferated, escaping the control of the bureaucratic and security apparatus.

The history of the accident of Yokadouma is thus the history of a "colonial scandal." The expression must be taken as an oxymoron, however, in the sense that a colony functions precisely as a site of exception that renders inoperative —by definition, one might say—any apparatus that might allow people to speak out, to accuse, to make reference to shared values, or to reach unanimity with respect to judgment and punishment, in other words, the very apparatus needed to define (and to participate in producing) a scandal and, at the same time, a public sphere.[4] If scandal, as its etymology ("stumbling block") suggests, is a "contradiction made public and visible to all, . . . a public fact, troubling and contradictory, that poses an obstacle to collective belief, and thereby sows dissent," according to Damien de Blic and Cyril Lemieux,[5] then its eruption is not inevitable, particularly not in a colonial situation. The history of Lomidinization opens a window onto the "painstaking work"[6] that produces affairs and scandals (through public condemnation) or buries them (by confining them within the parameters of a technical incident).

Scandals are privileged objects of historical investigation; they are *revelatory* of ordinary norms and relations of power, which are suddenly made explicit and questionable, and they are *foundational moments*—tests—from which institutions, positions, beliefs, and practices emerge altered.[7] Modern scandals are also bureaucratic and documentary phenomena: sensitive files. Studying scandals thus requires new ways of relating to archives, which might be characterized, borrowing from Ann Stoler, as "ethnographic." This makes archives no longer just sources, in and from which one discovers and extracts revelations, but also subjects. The very logics of archival production, classification, destruction, and conservation contribute to the definition and resolution of affairs, scandals, and accidents, according to how they are defined.[8]

The accident of Yokadouma was thus a matter of paper: a series of files was created precisely because of the threat of scandal in Paris and in Yokadouma, where telegrams, reports, letters, index cards, notes, delivery slips, and acknowledgments of receipt crossed paths and piled up. By engaging with these archives, following Stoler, through not only their content but also their form, it is possible to escape the reading that the reports seek to impose: the story of a technical incident resolved by colonial reason and strength, which follows the path of officials as they decipher clues, come to conclusions, and reaffirm their power. "If colonial documents reflected the supremacy of reason," Stoler suggests, "they also recorded an emotional economy manifest in disparate understandings of what was imagined, what was feared, what was witnessed, and what was overheard."[9] In the marginal annotations, in the repetition of formulaic statements and chronologies, in the juxtaposition of documents, gaps, and crossed-out words, the management of the accident of Yokadouma can be read other than as a deployment of rational knowledge. The handling of the events also put into practice a more fragile and nuanced, but also a more anxious colonial political art, aimed at negotiating appeasement and obtaining silence.

The disaster indeed perturbed the affective relations that defined and justified colonial domination: that is, the benevolence of the colonizers, exemplified by their medical services, and the affection given in return by the colonized. "Here, the native is content: he eats well, he is dressed, he understands our civilizing efforts, in a word: he loves us"—these are the lines Céline gave to a tired colonial doctor as he returned from Africa in the early 1930s.[10] The scandal of Lomidinization reveals the affective insecurity of a dying colonialism: it provides a glimpse of the fear that took hold of its agents, who were taken by surprise and at a loss in the face of Cameroonians' indignation and unanticipated ability to both articulate their outrage and put forward an analysis of the accident that upset the sequence generated by the official inquiry. The incident destabilized the order of things, knowledge, and values; it made emotion into a political language, used to voice and share indignation but also to appease and muffle it. In Yaoundé and in the Mbimou villages on the road to Yokadouma, the situation was resolved by shows of affection.

The Looming Scandal

When on the morning of November 15, Dr. Cauvin, the head of the SHMP, received the first telegram of alert from Yokadouma, his first reaction was anger: How could the chief regional officer have transmitted such sensitive information without encrypting the telegram to make it secret? Cauvin immediately made his way to the Directorate of Political and Administrative Affairs in order to, he said, using an administrative euphemism, "express his astonishment upon receiving a *plain-text* message containing such serious and as of yet unconfirmed news, likely to be exploited in the current session of the ATCAM."[11] The Assemblée territoriale du Cameroun (Territorial Assembly of Cameroon), which was made up of representatives of the Cameroonian people, settlers, and the administration, was indeed scheduled to meet that very day.

The establishment in 1946, as mandated by the Constitution of the Fourth Republic and of the Union française, of the ATCAM (which then took on various names) was part of postwar colonial reform. Colonial parliamentary life in the 1950s, where all future members of independent Cameroon's political elite cut their teeth, reflected broader nationalist political struggles. The UPC made its mark on the parliamentary process not by its effective presence in the assembly—indeed, the party was de facto excluded from the electoral process—but because its rejection became a condition for entry into the political profession. As Achille Mbembe has shown, submission to the colonial system, or at least the performance of submission, was a political resource in pre-independence Cameroon. In 1954, just when the parliamentary session was about to open, tension was building: High Commissioner André Soucadaux, a socialist, and his chief of staff, Georges Spénale, made it a priority of their administration to strike back, by means of police surveillance and harassment, against the UPC. Meanwhile, the UPC was gaining in popularity, thanks to its charismatic and determined leaders, who were capable of putting a radical social critique as well as a narrative of emancipation and national liberation into words and action. In November 1954, French colonialism in Cameroon hesitated between reform and repression.[12]

Cauvin no doubt thought the city was already agitated enough, and the medical campaigns difficult enough, and deemed it wise to avoid putting such dramatic topics—which, moreover, might yet turn out to be unfounded—within opponents' reach. The military doctor evidently did not appreciate the carelessness of the chief regional officer in sending an unencrypted message and asked for this "to be brought to his attention,"[13] using the polite language of the administration.

Meanwhile in Yokadouma, on that same morning of the fifteenth, Chief Regional Officer Gilbrin, "on the alert,"[14] had the postal clerk send a similar telegram, again in plain text, to apprise the High Commission of the events. The following morning, Gilbrin sent another plain-text telegram to the authorities to report "sixteen deaths and eighty gangrenes confirmed."[15] Spénale responded by coded telegram. The following was the *first official reaction* of the French Republic to the deaths in Yokadouma:

REGRET UNFORTUNATE PUBLICITY [YOU] HAVE GIVEN THIS AFFAIR THAT [YOU] SHOULD HAVE REPORTED TO ME BY CONFIDENTIAL CHANNEL IN CODE WHILE AWAITING CONCLUSION OF PUBLIC HEALTH INQUIRY[16]

This first response, written while the head of the SHMP was on his way to investigate in Yokadouma, ascribed, from the outset, the specific status of an "affair" to a series of deaths. The telegram was stamped "confidential" in red; all subsequent correspondence and reports also would be classified as confidential, and all further telegrams sent by the chief regional officer and by officials who traveled to Yokadouma would be "in code." However, as the telegram from the High Commission suggested, it was already too late—an affair, by definition, is not confidential. What "unfortunate publicity" had the news from Yokadouma received?

On the afternoon of November 15, the accident of Yokadouma had already slipped into the public arena. Gilbrin's first telegram had leaked after arriving at the High Commission; it reached René Mindjos, Yokadouma's elected counselor to the ATCAM. In the evening, when the Assemblée territoriale met for a long extraordinary session to debate the budget, a rumor circulated. Deputies passed the telegram around, and all of Yaoundé, so to speak, soon was talking about the deaths in Yokadouma. Around 11 p.m., as a discussion about the construction of a maternity clinic was underway, André-Marie Mbida, one of the rising stars of the ATCAM who also sat on the Assemblée consultative (Consultative Assembly) of the Union française in Paris, insisted on speaking:

> Mr. Mbida: Mr. Speaker, for some time, there is a treatment that has been applied here; it is a preventive treatment against sleeping sickness. It has already caused harm in this very region. Here, in the April session, I had drawn the attention of the Government, but today, M. Mindjos showed me a telegram by which he was informed that there have been several victims following, I believe, administration of this remedy. I am surprised that a drug that kills people is being used, and that instead of searching for the causes of this hazard, it continues to be used.
>
> Mr. Speaker: I do believe—despite the soundness of your observations—I do believe that the health services cannot use this drug, knowing that this drug kills people, because the nurses as well as the doctor who use it are directly responsible. The telegram that you speak of did indeed arrive and everyone is waiting for confirmation. I believe that an inquiry has been promptly launched to do so, and I thus think that it would be more prudent not to immediately appraise the situation and to wait for the result of the investigation.[17]

Mbida was a prominent figure in the assembly who, like other *évolués* (members of the educated or "assimilated" elite), had become a professional politician over the space of only a few years.[18] A protégé of the doctor, missionary, and minister Louis-Paul Aujoulat, Mbida was a former seminarian who had built a reputation as a formidable and ruthless orator and as a spearhead of the opposition to the UPC, yet he remained unpredictable in his position toward the French authorities.[19]

The Speaker of the Assemblée territoriale, Paul Soppo Priso, was not caught off guard by Mbida's intercession because he had been informed of the deaths. An ally of High Commissioner Soucadaux and his chief of staff and affiliated, like them, with the SFIO (the French Section of the Workers' International, a socialist political party), he was, by his position and personal wealth, the preeminent African in the Cameroonian political arena, playing the subtle role of "moderate nationalist."[20] He thus called Mbida, who was known for making dramatic declarations to the assembly, back to reason. But Mbida, who was testing the waters of a more vigorous critique of the French administration that would secure his political success, insisted.

A few months earlier in Eton country, Mbida's home region and political stronghold, there had been a few deaths,[21] while in the area of Yaoundé itself, Beaudiment's trials of Spécia's new Lomidine preparations had also caused some problems. The most recent deaths were not Lomidine's first, and Mbida remarked, alluding to the Stalinon scandal that had just shaken the metropole, that these calming calls to trust in the investigation were unconvincing: "The case [of the previous accidents with Lomidine] had been brought to the attention of the doctor in charge at the time. No serious investigation was conducted. But, I'd like to point out that, for example for Stalinon, there were very serious investigations. . . . Here, we think it enough to say that the nurse made a mistake."[22]

Soppo Priso now called for greater restraint: "Before taking a position, we must wait for the results [of the] investigation. I think this is wise and cautious, and we should not start attacking the Health Services before knowing what happened."[23] Another prominent political figure, Charles Assalé, backed him up from his seat. Assalé was a nurse by profession, who graduated at the top of the first class of the Ayos nursing school (founded by Jamot, which resulted in graduates being nicknamed "Jamotains"). Also affiliated with the socialist group, he kept his distance from radical nationalism:

Mr. Assalé: This is a technical question that exceeds the competence of the Assembly, and I think we can trust the Service in question, to give it time to shed light on the matter. . . . Perhaps the dose was too high, or the product was expired. Thus I ask my colleague Mbida to be more discerning in his affirmations by giving the Health Service time to do its research.

Mr. Mbida: What are you calling discerning[?] I pointed out that there were deaths.

Mr. Assalé: What I mean is to not be so definitive. We have to wait for the investigation to be done, and I do not think you can do it yourself.

Mr. Mbida: Nor you, you're not a doctor.

Mr. Assalé: Me neither, which is exactly why I am not speaking out.[24]

It was a lively exchange; synopses would mention "passionate interventions."[25] Other delegates joined the argument, which became confused. It took the Speaker's full standing to calm things down, and reports would praise his moderating action. While insisting on the need for an investigation, Soppo Priso closed the debate by reminding the assembly of the (colonial) epistemology to which they should all adhere and which justified keeping the events a state secret, as desired by the administration: "The reason we did not want to make the news official is because we deemed it necessary to act cautiously, for if the causes of this accident do not come from this drug, if the news got out too widely, Africans would come to mistrust this drug and no one would ever want to be treated with it."[26]

By putting an end to Mbida's outburst, the Speaker gave himself a way of resuming the budget debate on the meeting's agenda. As for placating Mbida, the administration, and "Africans," the work had only just begun.

Documentary Fever

The evening of November 15 was a paradoxical moment: just as the news was made public, the administration tried to keep it secret.

"Confidentialization" thus played a performative role: the administration was trying to convince itself that there was no reason to make a fuss about the accident of Yokadouma. Yet at the same time, it was seized by a documentary urge that clearly expressed the extent to which the stir caused by the events, of which the administration had just witnessed an obvious example in the assembly's discussions, was just as worrying as its public health impact. On the morning of November 16, by admonishing in a telegram its representative in Yokadouma and by making the decision to dispatch an inspector of administrative affairs, the colonial authorities demonstrated that they were dealing with a potential crisis: the technical management of the catastrophe was to be paired with an anxious endeavor to control its publicity.

In his first "confidential" telegram, sent on November 16, the chief regional officer of Yokadouma acknowledged the political dimension of the accident:

> I found out unofficially that the UPC and a few counselors of the ATCAM intend to come to Yokadouma at the end of the week. Because of the very serious health conditions following the anti-trypanosomiasis vaccination[s] that have caused, since Sunday, 16 deaths and many cases of serious complications, it would be preferable to avoid a popular meeting that could stir up regrettable unrest. I would thus be very grateful if you could dissuade, if possible, the ATCAM delegation from coming to Yokadouma at the present moment.[27]

The UPC's name had been dropped in; it would undoubtedly be heard by the government in Yaoundé, which was obsessed with the nationalist party and may have been put on guard by previous accidents. In the afternoon, Gilbrin wrote again and emphasized the "importance of [his previous] telegram" because "a resurgence of unrest is always possible although improbable."[28] Thus, the catastrophe of Yokadouma was defined, just hours after the uproar at the ATCAM, by the threat of scandal and by its potential to become a significant resource for the opposition movement. This should not be interpreted only as a product of the remote influence of political context on a technical and public health problem: the UPC was actively summoned by the affair's protagonists. In other words, the political context was constructed by the controversy itself, as microhistorical studies have shown in many other cases.[29]

Scandal exists by anticipation: the documentary frenzy reflects the magnitude of officials' anxiety. Most obviously, there was Ansellem's panic; the hastiness of the chief regional officer, who would need to apologize in his report for not having encrypted his initial missives; and the looming shadow of the UPC. And threats could come from anywhere, even after the affair was resolved: on December 8, for example, one of the nurses in charge of treating cases of gangrene at the kilometer 36 "treatment center" disappeared. The entire local population and Yokadouma's regional guards were mobilized to search with difficulty through dense forest for the nurse; Batouri's police officer investigated, while the high commissioner followed the case. What were the authorities worried about: a fugue state, vengeance, abandoned patients? The case was solved on December 12: the nurse had gone hunting and said he got lost. The officials breathed a sigh of relief, yet they attached all correspondence on this incident to the Lomidine file.[30] As fear took over, everything became relevant: the authorities no longer knew what they should disregard.

The hierarchies of credibility and of knowledge were inverted, as the assembly debates showed: Mbida and other counselors knew about Lomidine and its recurring accidents, while Assalé, in his response to them, spontaneously evoked tryparsamide, which had caused the Bafia accident in 1931. Their own memories of sleeping sickness control allowed them to summon the past with greater accuracy than the higher-ups at the head of the health service and the SHMP, who were replaced every four years. Those who had knowledge were no longer the doctors.

Cameroonians knew how to work comparisons: by evoking Stalinon—an anti-infective drug commercialized by a small firm based in the Paris region, which, as was exposed beginning in July 1954, caused about a hundred deaths in France—Mbida hit the nail on the head. The Stalinon affair, the first big postwar public health scandal, motivated in late 1954 a judicial inquiry and public debates that, beyond the question of the firm's liability, led to an indepth reexamination of the French system of drug monitoring and regulation.[31] Mbida seemed to know the affair well: he was close to Aujoulat, the French minister of health at the time of the Stalinon scandal. Why, in the case of Stalinon, had there been "very serious investigations"? And why, here, was it considered adequate to state "the nurse made a mistake"? With just a few words, André-Marie Mbida put his finger on one of the fundamental contradictions of colonial medicine, indeed of colonialism itself: the lives (and deaths) of the colonizers and those of the colonized did not have the same worth, and this inequality was, on the one hand, obviously organized by the colonial system, and was, on the other hand, wholly inconsistent with the republican ideals with which French domination identified. The principles of the republic versus republican colonialism—this clash could trip up a whole world.

Officials' anxiety was exacerbated by the fact that several doctors and nurses, both French and Cameroonian, held seats in the Assemblée territoriale, while there were also doctors among the UPC's leadership—indeed, the figure of the doctor-politician, of which Aujoulat was an example, was a familiar one in Cameroonian politics.[32] At that time, the UPC's president was Félix-Roland Moumié, an African doctor who had trained in Ayos and Dakar.[33] His work was exemplary, yet he was kept under close surveillance by the administration and transferred to ever more remote government postings. Conditions were ripe for a technical incident to turn into a political issue.

Threatened by its own technicians, the biopolitical state was growing nervous, to echo Nancy Rose Hunt's analysis of the Belgian Congo.[34] Although the toll of the catastrophe seemed to have stabilized, who knew where the affair would end, symbolically or geographically? Telegrams were sent to New York to brief the French delegation to the United Nations about the accident.[35] Indeed, the UPC had made the United Nations its main international forum, speaking out in New York against French colonialism in Cameroon on a regular basis. There was, no doubt, fear that questions would be asked publicly about the matter in Yokadouma.

The reports' release and the elucidation of the cause of the accident barely relieved the tension. On November 19, the Public Information Service published, on the basis of the first reports, a press release entitled "The Region of Yokadouma Mourns," which was reprinted in an Agence France-Presse dispatch. The Belgian doctors at the Ministry of Colonies in Brussels became aware of the news. The dispatch was handed around and annotated:

> Serious matter! unfortunately there is no detail on the kind of treatment. 11.24.54 [signed Duren]

> It is essential that the *cause* of these accidents be known, to avoid other tragedies. Could we not *discretely* ask Vaucel to tell us what is going on? Or should the BPITT in Léo[poldville] be alerted? 11.25.54 [signed Dr. De Brauwere]

> I would prefer to first get the opinion of Dr. Rhodain, who I can probably see next Tuesday. 11.26.54 [signed Duren]

> That is, indeed, wiser. Reviewed [signed Dr. De Brauwere].[36]

Words were underlined as if whispered; the written dialogue was anxious. Discretion was needed to find out more about the affair, news of which had only just arrived via the press. What was to be done? Should they raise the alarm, attempt to find out more from the French, or ask the advice of a veteran, Dr. J. Rhodain, a paragon of Belgian tropical medicine? Even in Brussels there was fear. But of what, they were not sure.

Demonstrating Affection

Relegated to the role of a looming threat, the UPC never intervened directly; to my knowledge, the party did not make public use of the incident, despite having often been associated with rumors about colonial medicine.[37] The UPC acted through its absence by enhancing, as a contrast, the political attractiveness of conciliatory positions. Emotion was not just a feature of the condescending characterization of the "African villager's" reaction, it was also a register of political action that entailed a performance and the instrumentalization of mourning and reconciliation.

In the late afternoon of November 18, Colonel-Doctor Vaisseau, the director of the Service de la santé publique du Cameroun (Public Health Service of Cameroon), attended an extraordinary session of the Assemblée territoriale. He came armed with the latest telegram from Yokadouma, which had, a few hours earlier, given him the first reassuring news: the doctors were hard at work, the patients were recovering, and the investigation was pointing toward the hypothesis of the defective filter. As promised following the debates of November 15, there was to be a presentation by the administration on the situation in Yokadouma. Invited by the Speaker of the assembly, Dr. Vaisseau delivered a solemn speech:

> Mr. Speaker, Gentlemen counselors, news of the dramatic accidents that just occurred in the region of Boumba-Ngoko during a [Lomidinization] session elicited dismay and distress at the Direction de la santé publique. Personally, I am moved, more touched than I can express. I think that, in this very painful affair, there is no space for any kind of criticism of our methods and their effectiveness. There is space [only] for collective emotion, emotion shared by all, you and us together, and that must find us clasped together, shoulder to shoulder.[38]

The tone in which the colonel spoke defused from the outset any attack that might have been brewing in the ranks of the assembly. The facts of the problem were, in just a few words, reversed; the accident was no longer a topic of conflict or controversy, but was instead a catalyst for solidarity between the administration and its Cameroonian constituents, who were united in suffering.

The next part of Vaisseau's speech was a display of the service's greatness. Vaisseau specified that the investigation had begun with the departure "by special airplane" of the head of the SHMP. He promised "harsh" sanctions and provided technical explanations of the conditions and causes of the accident. Vaisseau also spoke for Mindjos, the counselor accompanying the investigators in Yokadouma, who was said to have expressed "his full satisfaction." Vaisseau added that the incriminating samples were already on their way to the Institut d'hygiène (Institute of Hygiene) of Douala, the best laboratory in the country, and then he closed his presentation by paying tribute to the commitment of the doctors at the scene. The subsequent discussion clarified technical issues relating to the incident—the "planter's filter" and spores thus entered the assembly. Also emphasized was the "firm and unequivocal" commitment of the administration to "shed light on the entire matter" and to make public the judicial inquiry's conclusions. Finally, exceptional financial support was unanimously approved.

Above all, the addresses to the assembly made a show of shared suffering. The Speaker's first reaction was "to receive this news with great pain and to honor the unfortunate victims." The assembly also observed a "minute of reflection." The Speaker continued, acknowledging the emotion expressed by Vaisseau: "Mr. Director, we were also, like you, very moved, but also, your presentation was full of emotion. We are fully aware that the Service de santé was deeply affected by this unfortunate accident. Given that the inquiries are ongoing, the Assemblée territoriale asks for only one thing: that the administration use every means available to stop accidents."[39]

Soppo Priso went on to remind his audience, as if to better convince himself, of one of the fundamental postulates of modernizing colonialism, that is, the infallibility of medical goodwill and reason—and its corollary, the unfortunate accident: "We know, Mr. Director, that the Service de santé cannot, in any way, be held under suspicion, quite the contrary; the very fact that 3,000 individuals were treated proves that the Service de santé is doing its job and that it is an accident such as might happen anywhere; just recently, despite the highly technical procedures of the metropole, we saw a more or less analogous case."[40]

Here, Soppo Priso could show off his political skill—indeed, he had built his career on a carefully staged yet subtle submission to colonial power:

> I am taking this opportunity, while we have you with us, and I believe the circumstances are fitting, for we do not want you to take our observations as specific criticism of the Service de santé. I am taking this opportunity to pay you, on behalf of the Assembly, our most respectful compliments for the decoration you have just been awarded. We have learned that you have just been made an officer of the Legion of Honor. We truly believe that you have earned it by your highly devoted services that you have given to Cameroon, and continue to give (*applause*). We thus bid you be assured that our full sympathies are with you in this painful ordeal, which is the ordeal not only of the Service de santé, but of the whole territory.[41]

"Everything to be said was said," added the government commissioner to this rather strange closing to the parliamentary controversy about Yokadouma. The switch of perspective was now complete: in the end, it was to the health service that the assembly addressed its condolences, and the debate on the catastrophe was concluded by a reaffirmation of trust in colonial doctors' enterprise. The only public confrontation relating to this affair—which is probably the most violent iatrogenic accident in African history—thus ended in unanimous applause for the figure who, in principle, bore the most responsibility. This shows, one might say, the baroque nature of responsibility that prevailed in the Cameroonian colony. A critique of medical action seems, in this context, to have been extremely difficult to formulate, as was clear to counselor Jean Mabaya, who made an attempt, after this solemn celebration of the great doctor, to get back to the issue of accidents. "I am not criticizing the practitioners," he felt the need to declare in a conciliatory opening, before drawing attention to the reoccurrence of accidents during Lomidinization campaigns, pointing out that there had also been deaths in his district of Abong-Mbang in the Haut-Nyong. Faith in public health and its methods thus endured as the necessary preamble, and conclusion, to any audible discourse on the catastrophe.

Conciliation was also orchestrated in Yokadouma by putting on display both the docility of the population and the magnanimity of the administration and, concretely, by seeing to the rapid distribution of substantial "financial help." Just days after the accident, reports were already commending the part played by canton chiefs (that is, the Cameroonian collaborators of the administration) in calming down the situation. The letter these chiefs wrote to the high commissioner on November 19 to claim indemnities indicates they were aware of the price of their conciliatory attitude. "We cried without making a palaver," they recalled in their request.

Mr. High Commissioner,
Mr. Attorney General,

We, Mpega Martin, chief of Mbimou canton and Wissambo Awoui, chief of Yanghere [*sic*] canton in the region of the Boumba-Ngoko, place ourselves in your hands to ask for justice and compensation.

The last Lomidinization tour to visit our cantons caused the death of 25 persons. Some are still at death's door and will soon die.

We want that justice be done and that those responsible be punished proportionally to the misfortune that befalls us.

For the widows, the children, the family members of the deceased, we ask for indemnities of justice.

We count on you heavily as we face the catastrophe that just happened, for all we did was to carry out the law that made Lomidine compulsory and that brought us death.

Our chief regional officer, before this situation of general bereavement, promised us that justice would be done. We trust him and that is why we all have cried without making a palaver.

Mr. High Commissioner, Mr. Attorney General, bring justice quickly to this affair.[42]

Initially, the amounts proposed for compensation payments were modest: the chief regional officer at first suggested 2,000 francs per deceased and 1,000 francs per individual with serious complications, for a total of 175,000 francs. The high commissioner responded with an assignment of 500,000 francs; this generosity reveals the importance that was given, in high places, to resolving this affair.[43] An additional million francs was approved by the assembly, which resulted in a considerable sum to be distributed to victims and their families in January 1955.[44] An eyewitness who stayed in Yokadouma after taking part in the SHMP's "rescue mission" gives an account that hints at what this process of compensation might have entailed:

And then we were ordered to go at once to treat the population. And then we compensated all the deaths, I don't remember how much they were compensated. And after that, the guys they would nearly have finished off, those who were just injured, it was disgusting, it was really . . . the behavior of the local population was despicable. They would have nearly finished killing those people to get their money. It's true that money was scarce at the time. . . .

You weren't met with stones? People didn't protest?

No, as soon as they were promised compensation, it's amazing what a huge effect that had. They had never seen so much money. I think that they got, for each deceased, 150,000 or 200,000 francs.[45]

It is difficult to judge the truth of what is described in this witness's account. Yet it is clear that the financial compensation brought a jolt, both material and symbolic, to this peripheral region. André Soucadaux, Cameroon's "socialist-conservative" high commissioner from 1949 to 1954, had indeed made a hallmark of such acts of largesse; today, we would call it corruption. By adding to official ceremonies—where medals or promotions were awarded to low-ranking chiefs and clerks—the practice of handing out money or drinks, the French colonial administration, including its health service, participated in establishing what would remain a crucial mechanism for the postcolonial political elite: the ostentatious purchase of public peace. The shower of francs that rained on several villages of the Boumba-Ngoko in January 1955, or the vulgar motivations of the African chiefs evoked in accounts of the Lomidinization campaigns in Saa, are certainly examples of this mode of government.

The affair of Yokadouma was concluded with demonstrations of reciprocal affection. In late December, the Cameroonian Medal of Merit was awarded to the African doctor Théodore Botétémé, to Captain-Doctor Constant, and to the "chiefs of the harshly tested cantons."[46] At the Institut d'hygiène in Douala, the results were inconclusive, and all the samples were sent, in the hope of an ultimate moment of microbiological truth, to the Institut Pasteur in Paris. The results from Paris were, the chief regional officer mentioned in one of his political reports, "awaited impatiently" in Yokadouma.[47]

Archiving as Burial

Achille Mbembe, in an apt meditation on archives that resonates with his own study of the UPC, wrote, "archives . . . constitute a type of sepulchre," an apparatus aiming to "ensure that the dead do not stir up disorder in the present": "Archiving is a kind of interment, laying something in a coffin, if not to rest, then at least to consign elements of that life which could not be destroyed purely and simply."[48]

Archiving in the Yokadouma case followed close on the heels of bereavement ceremonies and the public display of shared grief. On December 2, 1954, the High Commission requested, by confidential note, that the Direction d'affaires politiques et administratives "put together a very complete file on the events in Yokadouma including a copy of the debates at the Assemblée territoriale and the reports of the various figures who wrote about the topic."[49] The folder containing the file that was created bears several annotations: "Vaccinations," "Accidents during the Lomidinization Campaigns—November 1954," and "Boumba-Ngoko Region/Yokadouma Subdivision/Incidents/Lomidinization." This file, to which was added some later correspondence on the evolution of the situation in Yokadouma, became file 3 AC 1871 of the National Archives of Cameroon; it was renamed during an inventory "Boumba-Ngoko (Cameroon), Lomidinization 1954–1956. Does treatment with Lomidine carry risks? Case of the Boumba-Ngoko 1954–1956." This is not the file of a scandal or an affair, but of a medical case and accidents.

This file, which holds the entire set of telegrams in and out of Yokadouma,

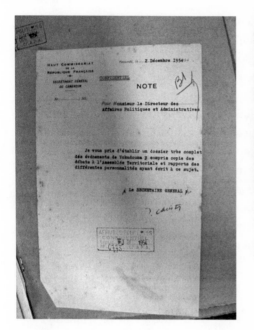
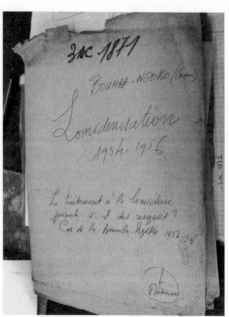

Note from the high commissioner requesting the creation of an archival file on the incident, December 2, 1954; and the cover of the 3AC 1871 file. National Archives, Yaoundé, Cameroon.

copies of all the reports, and the verbatim transcription of the debates at the Assemblée territoriale, made it easy to tell the story as I have. These records owe as much to the fear of the administration as to its political calculations, its will to both anticipate the scandal and to bury the file, in the literal sense of the term: to ensure that this affair was over. For the High Commission, the act of archiving was indeed a means of keeping ghosts silent, of gathering the remains left by the dead of Yokadouma to counteract "the possibility, always there, that left to themselves, they might eventually acquire a life of their own,"[50] to prevent the past from remaining present in other forms: as scandal, memory, rumor.

"In conclusion, this sad affair . . . could be restored to the proportions of an unfortunate accident"[51]—these were the words that closed the official report of the high commissioner of the French Republic in Cameroon, sent to Paris on December 31. The whole purpose of the colonial administration, including its nurses and archivists, is surely apparent in this shortcut.

Tangoulou

It is 7 p.m. Joseph has cooked up a nice little dinner in honor of the doctor, who for the occasion has taken out a good bottle of Saint-Émilion: vermicelli soup, roast chickens, potatoes sautéed with onions, and local fruits. In addition, we will attend, invited by the Kongo chief, the dances that have been organized for tonight, when the big drums will be taken out. . . . [The] dances are starting and will continue until about midnight.

The next morning, we leave Vindza at eight for the planned testing session. Around 1 p.m., on the way back . . . we meet a man on the road; beside him lies a young woman who is about twenty-six years old, her name is Tangoulou.

Asked, her husband, Milandou, informs us that she received, with the residents of the village, an injection of Lomidine and that, for three days, has complained of pain in her right buttock, at the site of injection. . . .

Upon examination, the whole buttock is, indeed, edematous, presenting an induration deep below which, under the mass of the gluteals, palpation reveals crepitus. The pain is intense, mobility is nearly fully impaired. The general state is very altered, the pulse is weak, irregular.

Tangoulou is transported at once to the dispensary of Vindza. Upon arrival, very marked signs of gangrenous toxemia are noted. The pulse is weaker and weaker, with muffled and irregular heartbeats and cooling of the extremities. . . . At 2:30 p.m., the patient falls into syncope; she is reanimated, but she dies, fully conscious, at three of an acute form of gas gangrene in the right buttock, probably following an injection that was not rigorously aseptic.

. . .

The village is in turmoil. There is a lot of noise and endless palavering. The villagers have gathered and are speaking in determined voices. A young woman is dead and it is of our making. Of my making, I should say, because for the natives, the only person in charge is the European chief of the team. . . .

There will be no dancing this evening in the square and, if the drums beat, it is to pass the message, to inform about the death of Tangoulou.

The Kongo chief understands very well what happened. He is trying to calm the villagers, to temper the passion in their discussions. He asks us also not to go out too much in the village, to remain in the guest hut. He will do all he can to calm things down. As a precaution, for the night, we have blocked the door of the hut with tin trunks, which will make noise if someone tries to enter.

F. Gauthier, *Lutte contre la trypanosomiase et la lèpre en Afrique 1953–1960. Mission d'une équipe médicale mobile de prospection du Service général d'hygiène et de prophylaxie* (Éditions des Écrivains, Paris, 2000), 101–2, 105–6.

CHAPTER NINE

The Misfires of the Imperial Machine

For me, it's a question of method: you have to begin from the sand caught in the gears. If you take rules as your starting point, you run the risk of falling into the illusion that they work, and then miss the anomalies. But if you begin from the anomalies, the dysfunction, you will find rules there too, because they are implicated.

—Carlo Ginzburg, "De près, de loin. Entretien avec Philippe Mangeot," *Vacarme* (2002)

Nkoltang, Nola, Saa, Yokadouma, Goro—the accident of Yokadouma would not warrant a whole book were it not for the recurrence of similar Lomidinization accidents during the 1950s, adding up to a long list of "stupid deaths."[1] The documentary ordering of the catastrophe was also a way of ensuring its repetition: archiving as forgetting.

Historians of science have often been mesmerized by the "colonial machine," thus describing colonialism as a system of domination held up by science and reason.[2] How can we write history otherwise in order to reveal the machine's underbelly, its constitutive misfires and mediocrity? Certainly, we would need a new way of looking at archives: by reading between the lines, by reading against the grain of the projects and orders the documents contain. Or instead, we could take up Ann Stoler's call to follow the thread of the archive by reading it according to its own logics, along the grain: in other words, we can look, like an anthropologist in the field, not for what the archive hides or represses, but for what it *does*.[3]

By rereading in this way the stack of papers generated by the accident of Yokadouma, it becomes possible to understand how the machine of the colonial health service (dys)functioned, to understand how this institution of empire projected an image of a rational apparatus for managing humans, things, and information and, at the same time, projected another, indissociable image of an ineffective administration whose memory and coherence one would be wrong to overestimate. The tragedy thereby appears not so much as an anomaly but instead as a product of the pragmatic and rational norms that governed the practice of colonial medicine. If the accident of Yokadouma was a red-hot case that needed to be managed, it was also what Ben Kafka calls a Freudian "slip":[4] a bureaucratic catastrophe produced by the very logics of the machine designed to plan, document, and quantify the activities of Lomidinization campaigns. In the archives of the colonial health service, the file on the Yokadouma accident is juxtaposed with the files on virtually identical catastrophes—as if archiving were not so much a means of putting back in order, but rather a way of organizing the repetition of massacre.

The Archiving Machine

On November 17, 1954, the cabinet of the High Commission in Yaoundé alerted the Ministère de la France d'Outre-Mer, with the usual precautions:

TOP PRIORITY

CONFIDENTIAL—stop—

About twenty deaths are reported by chief regional officer YOKADOUMA which according to initial news appear linked to recent Lomidinization—stop—Medical reinforcements immediately dispatched as well as colonel doctor in chief of Mobile Hygiene Service and inspector of Administrative Affairs.

Will keep you informed results ongoing inquiry as well as any new information.[5]

Transmitted to the head office of the colonial health services, this telegram introduced the affair into the circuits of the French imperial state. Established within the Ministère de la France d'Outre-Mer, which had its buildings on the rue Oudinot in Paris, the office was a well-oiled apparatus for deploying expertise and decision making, where, year after year, a substantial number of documents were filed.[6] In contact with the Institut Pasteur in Paris, the head office was the nerve center of colonial medicine and was considered a highly prestigious posting for end-of-career colonial doctors; in 1954, following Marcel Vaucel's long tenure from 1944 to 1952, General-Doctor Robert (full name unknown) was in charge. The head office was a medical and military enclave within a ministerial bureaucracy; its entire set of archives was, in the early 1960s, taken over by an institute belonging to the army's health service, the École du Pharo in Marseille. This is where I consulted the documents in the early 2000s; the school's closure in 2013 began a new phase in the wanderings of this archival collection.

From November 17, 1954, all telegrams received about Yokadouma in the offices of the "sad hive"[7] on rue Oudinot were stamped with the requisite "confidential." In the "4th Office,"[8] documents were stamped again to confirm reception; they were then read and annotated by the general-doctor, stacked, paper clipped, and finally assembled in the latest "Trypanosomiasis" file. The traces of the incident of Yokadouma were thus interleaved among other documents in box 253 of the IMTSSA Archives in a subsection of the collection "Diseases and Parasites"—in other words, in the scientific archives, among manuscripts, reprints, and celebrations of Lomidinization authored by the leading trypanosomiasis experts of the colonial health corps.

The irony of this classification, which intertwines miracle with disaster, draws attention to the fact that archival form has a content of its own, which is revealing of what archiving "does." As in Yaoundé, where the high commissioner gave the order to archive when the catastrophe had barely been contained, the file created in Paris was not merely a record of state mobilization; it also participated in restoring order to the situation as much as the medical action per se. The file I examined testifies to a set of hierarchical relations, the "work of the state on itself,"[9] in which the control of doctors and administrators—who risked their careers if they made a mistake in their telegrams or failed to find the right formulation—was also at stake. And so we should not see archives as transcripts of how administrations already worked, that is, of an already-there mode of administrative operation, nor should we take at face value the coherence and power they document. Archiving functions as a fiction, as the "stories that states tell themselves."[10]

One archival fiction was emergency. In Paris, the initial alerting telegram, received on November 17, was annotated with a time of reception accurate to the minute: "at 11:40."[11] Meanwhile in Cameroon, more than three days had gone by since the first cases were reported (most people, to put it bluntly, had finished dying); it had been more than ten hours since the SHMP rescue truck had left Yaoundé, and it was now rattling along in the dust toward Yokadouma. But from the moment the first message was labeled "top priority"—the highest level of administrative urgency—the emergency was systematically evoked in all correspondence circulated during the two weeks of the affair. At the end of December, as the cabinet of the High Commission in Yaoundé was putting the finishing touches on its summary report for the ministry, its office sent yet another "extremely urgent" letter to obtain the SHMP's stamp: the handwritten

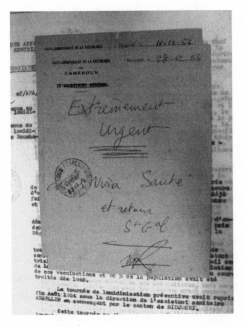

Anonymous handwritten note "Extremely Urgent" on the letterhead of the High Commission of Cameroon, December 28, 1954. 3 AC 1871, National Archives, Yaoundé, Cameroon.

injunction was underlined four times.[12] Another archival fiction was secrecy. Every document assembled in Paris was "confidential," even an inquiry from the Ministère de la santé et de la population (Ministry of Health and Population), although it was mentioned that the ministry knew about the accident from the Agence France-Presse, which had broadcast a dispatch in its daily news bulletin on Cameroon.[13]

There is a striking disconnect between, on the one hand, this ritualization of secrecy and of emergency at the ministry and, on the other hand, the publicity and actual rhythm of events in Yokadouma. The "public secret" is a classic paradox: as Stoler shows in her study of a "colonial affair" in Java, the secret in this case clearly did not apply to the facts referred to in the documents, but rather to the indecision, contradictions, disagreements, tensions, and emotions of officials.[14] Just as urgency was part of a more general attempt to abolish time and distance within the empire, the secret here was not the accident, but rather that the administration was paralyzed by fear.

The Action Machine

Nevertheless, the machine of the colonial Service de santé acted: the accumulation of information gave way to a cascade of decisions.

The diagnosis (gangrene caused by a contaminated solution) did not, it seems, come as a surprise to Parisian experts. Over the previous months, the use of powdered Lomidine had been questioned amid growing awareness of the high risks entailed by the practice of preparing solutions in water. When news of the accident of Yokadouma reached rue Oudinot, the first question to be posed was economic: How much would it cost to give up the powdered form and use industrially prepared Lomidine solution instead? For the answer, the head office turned to Henri de Marqueissac, a former colonial doctor who, after retiring, took the position of head of trypanosomiasis at Spécia. De Marqueissac was also one of the few veterans of the Mission Jamot who was still working; he was thus a "confrere" in the strongest sense of the term.

De Marqueissac's response relayed significant price differences between the Lomidine preparations marketed by Spécia: while Lomidine powder cost 80 francs per gram, the equivalent of ready-to-use solution sold in flasks cost 130 francs. De Marqueissac gave a projection for the Cameroonian case: substituting the solution for the powder would incur, based on 250,000 injections per year, an additional cost of 2 million metropolitan francs before taxes and shipping. In Cameroon, an agreement had just been passed in early November for the provision of 80 kilograms of Lomidine powder. De Marqueissac asked General-Doctor Robert: "Shall we maintain our order or change it for flasks of solution?"[15]

The economic dilemma was quickly settled. On December 3, Robert addressed a telegram, in plain text this time, to the high commissioners of the republic in the African colonies. In Dakar, Brazzaville, Yaoundé, and Lomé, an explicit order was received:

To [Department of] Public Health
Extemporaneous solution of Lomidine requires manipulation that can cause serious accidents STOP please firmly prohibit use of powder Lomidine STOP Only solution prepared by Spécia must be used STOP Detailed instructions to follow END France d'Outre-Mer[16]

Letters addressed to the governors followed, with a reminder of the terrible toll of the accident of Yokadouma. Even though "the product itself could not be incriminated, no more than could the principle of Lomidine chemo-prophylaxis," its powder form was to be abandoned despite being cheaper "by about 50%" than the readymade solution. "Economic factors cannot . . . be taken into consideration when it comes to potential accidents, which are always serious, since they have already cost a number of human lives."[17]

The directive was applied at once. Across AEF, Lomidinization was suspended. The federation's stocks of now useless Lomidine powder were substantial: the quantities scattered across its regions added up to more than 160 kilograms, enough for two years of chemoprophylaxis. It was a hard blow to the federation's already strained finances and hard, also, on Lomidinization statistics. The situation in AOF was not quite as complicated; there, the SGHMP had nearly stopped using Lomidine powder during the previous three years.[18]

Spécia facilities—in Vitry-sur-Seine, where the molecule was produced, and in Saint-Fons, where Lomidine was prepared and packaged—scrambled to adapt in just a few days. "Following the recent incidents in Cameroon—and even though our product was found to be absolutely free of blame—it has been decided to abandon the use of Lomidine in powder form and to use only solutions," announced the commercial department to the rest of Spécia's departments on December 6. They wondered: Should the firm "give satisfaction [to Cameroon] that very important client," which would require taking back its stocks of powder? Should they "stop the production of the 300 kg of isethionate [powder] in Vitry?"[19] The commercial department then decided: the Ministère de la France d'Outre-Mer had been unequivocal; they must get ready for massive orders of Lomidine solution.[20]

Orchestrated in Paris, the reaction was swift and firm. The organizational charts of the Services de santé coloniale were set in motion, stirred into action by directives from the "4th Office" on rue Oudinot to nurses touring the outer edges of French Africa. The Services d'hygiène et de prophylaxie could get back to work, and all could praise the "very beneficial effects" of the measure. In AEF, there was reassurance: "Battles, especially big ones, rarely go according to plan. AEF has benefited from the unfortunate experience of some neighbors, and thus managed to avoid any serious accidents. This has led to a dip in the statistics; this is nothing compared to the consequences that might have followed the accidents we have avoided."[21]

The file was closed. In mid-December 1954, General-Doctor Robert wrote up an "Information Card on the Topic of Trypanosomiasis Prophylaxis by

Lomidine—Accidents in Cameroon." Placed on the top of the archival pile, the memorandum was not addressed to anyone: what mattered in the act of recopying the narrative of the reports written in Cameroon was that the state told *itself* a story that was lucid and reassuring.

As for Spécia, the firm was getting ready to replace Lomidine powder with solution and, surely, to make additional profits.

Accidents as Stuttering

A grain of sand, however, snuck into the machinery resolving the problem of the accident of Yokadouma. It showed up in a confidential telegram, which was archived in Yaoundé. On November 22, 1954, the chief regional officer in Batouri, where Captain-Doctor Constant was back after a difficult week in Yokadouma, informed the High Commission: "the regional doctor in chief had brought to my attention that in December 1953, deaths similar to those of Yokadouma seem to have occurred in Libreville." While reading the telegram, the chief of staff annotated by hand: "Ask information Gabon for connection."[22] Such a connection was never made, and Constant's comment did not make it into the official analysis. Yet the information this telegram delivered was major: almost a year earlier, near Libreville in AEF, an accident similar to Yokadouma's in magnitude and causation had happened. This makes the catastrophe of Yokadouma come into view as a rerun, a repeat offense, a stutter. The affair had a precedent, and its bureaucratic management was informed by this fact—even if the precedent was addressed only through *active* ignorance, amnesia, or lack of comparison. And so, another facet of the imperial apparatus is unveiled: the archiving machine is also a forgetting machine.

Furthermore, Dr. Constant got the year wrong in his telegram. It was, in fact, in December 1952 that the "accidents of Nkoltang" took place—and that a "Nkoltang file" was opened.[23] As in Yokadouma, a "perfectly experienced" team, headed by a subaltern agent identified only as Sergeant Thomas, "an old hand at *la trypano*," had set out by truck to "Lomidinize a road"—specifically, the villages situated along the road between Libreville and Kango—over the course of about fifteen days. At the road's kilometer 30 point in the village of Nkoltang, three days after Lomidinization, a series of cases of gas gangrene was reported by the police, warranting the evacuation of forty-four individuals to the hospital at Libreville and causing a total of fourteen deaths. As in Yokadouma, the reaction of the colonial administration was demonstrative: first aid, penicillin, and gas gangrene antitoxin helped limit the fatality rate;

a "mission of inquiry" got to work in the very first days after the arrival "by air" of Colonel-Doctor André Lotte, the head of the SGHMP; a judicial investigation was opened; and the sergeant was put under "strict arrest." By the first week of January, Lotte, who happened to be a leading expert on Lomidinization, was already giving his conclusions, and he sent a circular to all the mobile team chiefs, urging them to "check the instructions" of their staff and to scrupulously follow official directives. As in Yokadouma, the final report addressed to Paris demonstrated that the cause of the gangrene in Nkoltang was the use of contaminated solution.

The accident of Nkoltang also got the imperial bureaucratic machine running full steam. Immediately upon receiving the first official report, rue Oudinot replied with a harsh letter, demanding a more thorough inquiry that was to be independent from the judicial investigation. "The account of the director of the SGHMP is not a proper report," retorted the director of the Services de santé coloniale, who went on to request, among other things, the names of all protagonists, the practical details of how the team operated, each nurse's role, an hour-by-hour account of the catastrophe and the emergency response, the batch numbers of the Lomidine that was used, and detailed descriptions of the clinical cases and the biological tests performed (the list went on for two pages). The response from the chief of staff to the high commissioner in Brazzaville, in April 1953, was a thick envelope with copies of the detailed reports on all clinical cases and on the autopsies and many tests conducted. Lotte included a new, more comprehensive report, appending a copy of the technical instructions given to the mobile teams; he concluded that the health assistant bore "full responsibility." Finally, the general secretary of the high commissioner himself signed a seven-page summary letter; it was a valiant endeavor of technopolitical "translation" that presented, rather didactically, every theoretically possible hypothesis for the contamination and then went on, playing detective, to rule them out one by one. "The concept of the source of contamination thus presents itself with a logic that comes close to evidence," he ended, putting the blame, in an "infinitely probable" way, on the preparation of the solution.

The accident of Nkoltang did not become an affair of state: in Gabon, there was no administrative inquiry or political debate. Confined to the bounds of medical expertise, the catastrophe of Nkoltang required less work in order to rebuild, after the fact, the cosmology and epistemology of the colonial world. The reports, of course, devoted a few lines to praising the "great alacrity" of response of the health services and self-congratulation on the fact that "the accidents did not have, on the popularity of chemoprophylaxis, the unfortunate repercussions that we might have feared." To clearly mark the boundaries of colonial rationality, the reports also conveyed, concerning "the natives," the possibility of the "criminal intervention of a third party, either in revenge (toward the operations or the patients), or for hatred of the method (superstition, prejudice)" as well as the "misguided actions of Lomidinized subjects following the shot (native remedies, scarification, application of local plasters on the injection site)" and even the difficulty of "accepting without reservation people's testimony about operations whose meaning and mechanism they do not fully grasp." The villagers had even mentioned "a setup by Cameroonians" on the health team, and they had been troubled by the fact that "the first victim [had] been the wife of the witch doctor," one doctor remarked in order to better emphasize, by way of contrast, the reliability of his own investigation. Still, on the whole, the accidents remained legible in the genre of the technical incident, in this case an incident that was especially astonishing in that it appeared, according to the reports, to have been virtually impossible. "It seems to be . . . an accidental unpredictable individual failing of a technician who until then had been perfect and whose altogether laudable past counts as an extenuating circumstance," the general secretary to the governor of Brazzaville concluded.

And so, in early 1953, the Nkoltang file was closed. In the offices of rue Oudinot, it joined—as a regrettable accident—a "Trypanosomiasis" file destined to grow thicker with the determined pursuit of Lomidinization campaigns.

The Forgetting Machine

In retrospect, that the same type of accident reoccurred only 1,000 kilometers away nearly two years later already testifies to a first "misfire" in how these incidents were understood: the specific riskiness of making up Lomidine solution was not identified, and the carelessness of the nurse-sergeant was accepted as the sole cause of the damage. "Routine lulls precaution," the director of Mobile Hygiene had explained;[24] therefore, a call to order appeared to be an adequate measure for preventing the recurrence of such accidents. Yet the problem was not limited to such retrospective considerations. Indeed, the investigators' conclusions seem to have been rendered inaudible, muddled by the persistent interference of contradictory discourses on the causes of the accident. An alternative interpretation had continued to circulate, particularly in official publications, despite being dismissed by the reports. In it, the focus was on patients' own responsibility; they were seen as guilty of dangerous "manipulations" after being injected. This hypothesis, taken up and repeated as an obvious fact, helped to cloud the comprehension of the accident, making the investigations' conclusions unintelligible.

An early instance of such an explanation arose in the account that Colonel-Doctor Lavergne (full name unknown), the director of public health in Gabon, addressed to the state prosecutor, in which, going against his own investigators' conclusions, he pointed the finger at "native customs."[25] Effortfully, he explained to the prosecutor how the gangrene might have been caused not by the inoculation of a germ, but rather by a mechanical or chemical attack on the muscles, for which the victims themselves were to blame. He went on to skillfully manipulate the contradictions of the contemporary scientific literature. Summoning "Professor Gosset's *Traité de pathologie chirugicale* [*Treatise of Surgical Pathologies*], whose authority no one can deny," Lavergne pointed out that even in the metropole under conditions of apparently perfect asepsis, isolated cases of gas gangrene following injections were not uncommon, particularly with drugs known to be "aggressive," which caused inflammation, even necrosis, at the site of injection.[26] Contemporary medicolegal experts held that gas gangrene could develop from a mere injury to muscles, even without inoculation of the bacillus. Then, Lavergne explained, injected subjects had added their fateful contribution: "Some individuals might, after the shot, have applied a traumatizing or caustic treatment at the point of inoculation (pressure, plaster, etc.). This [practice] was indeed reported . . . during previous Lomidinization tours."[27] The new theory absolved the health services while reinforcing a long-standing interpretation of the failures of the colonial medical enterprise: the detrimental action of "the natives."

This maneuver by the director of public health in his commitment to defend his service—even if it meant slightly twisting the findings of the investigations—would have been of little relevance if his interpretation had not, over the following months, been elevated to the status of an official conclusion. The venerable Gaston Muraz, for example, mentioned the Gabon accidents in one of his tributes to Lomidinization in early 1954, making a direct link between "indisputable septic errors" and the post-injection practices of "the natives." "If the contamination of the diamidine solution had been to blame, shouldn't it have resulted in thousands of [abscesses]?" he asked pointedly, cheerfully contradicting, despite citing, the "painstaking investigations."[28] Pierre Richet, his heir in AOF, restated this conclusion before the experts in the field gathered in Pretoria, South Africa, in September 1954: "The very thorough investigations conducted after these accidents nevertheless allow for the possibility that the victims may have been responsible for their own gangrene, the natives of this region having sometimes the deplorable habit of applying after injection, on the site of the shot, a sort of plaster made with . . . wet mud and mashed banana."[29] At least in Richet's case, it is hard to invoke senility or ignorance: Jacques Pépin, who provided me with a copy of this document, annotated in the margin: "He knew this was not true!"

The majority of reports then reiterated this interpretation, which posed an obstacle to understanding the accidents on a technical level—in addition to distorting the findings of the investigations. This is one of the conditions that allowed the disaster of Nkoltang to be repeated in Yokadouma.

Yet there is another, even more concerning fact about the administrative machine of the colonial health service: *none* of the expert assessments on the accident of Yokadouma, with the exception of Dr. Constant's comment, mentioned the precedent of Nkoltang. True, it is likely that the inquiries conducted in Yokadouma and the rapid decision to proscribe Lomidine in powder form in December 1954 were informed by knowledge of the previous accidents. It is also likely that mentioning Nkoltang would have been embarrassing, in which case the omission may have been intentional. Yet the archival juxtaposition, just a few files apart, of the meticulous accounts of both accidents speaks for itself; this does, indeed, signal a second misfire. It exposes the flip side of the imperial bureaucracy's show of force. At best, it reveals the mediocre quality of its archival mechanics: the apparent inefficiency in transmitting files, as a form of technical memory, between successors at the head of the Service de santé colonial. Worse, what is unmasked here is the capacity of the system to forget, even, one might say, to ensure its own amnesia.

"I Wonder How It Is That There Are Not More 'Hiccups'"

By following the thread of the archives, it becomes possible to understand how the repetition of accidents (that is, their serial forgetting) was actively organized. The old inspectors may have been amnesic, but Spécia certainly was not—the firm kept count of the accidents—nor were young bush doctors such as Yves Constant or Jacques Pierre Ziegler, for whom, even before Yokadouma,

Lomidinization accidents were a topic of conversation. Therefore, the repetition of catastrophes was made possible because of an active ignorance, an explicit will to not know.

Cases of gangrene recurred on a regular basis; Richet had even, in early 1954, compiled a list in one of his reports.[30] Spécia had reconsidered the use of Lomidine in powder form, given the apparent risks of preparing solution in the field. Thus, Henri de Marqueissac, a former Jamotain turned Spécia advisor, arranged in 1953 for an experiment to compare the advantages and drawbacks of the powder and solution forms of Lomidine. Jacques Pierre Ziegler, then posted in Chad, was put in charge of running it; he received instructions directly from de Marqueissac, along with a parcel of Lomidine.[31] Ziegler was not a typical expert: he was barely thirty years old, a civilian, meaning that he was not a member of the colonial corps, and he mastered both theory and practice. In May 1953, he was on his "9th semestral injection of Lomidine, since '48." That he was chosen by de Marqueissac, who knew the small world of *la trypano* inside out, was a form of anointment.

In early 1953, Ziegler tested, including *on himself*, various Lomidine preparations. As a "readymade" solution, the injection caused a "sharp, even very sharp pain," but "result[ed] in nearly no shock nor hypertension . . . no feeling of nausea, no sweating, no vertigo . . . while, with the solution prepared from distilled water, there [was] almost always (probably always) an unpleasant sensation that force[d] you to sit down for at least ten minutes." Ziegler even mentioned that in a European doctor he had Lomidinized, the sensation of numbness in the buttocks had lasted several months. His reply to de Marqueissac continued:

> Yet I think that the huge advantage of the readymade solution is not in relation to this issue. . . . In my opinion, the already prepared solution is highly preferable:
>
> 1. because its sterility is guaranteed ([a condition] that we are unfortunately never certain of having with solutions prepared by African nurses);
> 2. because its dosage is always accurate (while the solution made up in the bush has only an approximate percentage [of concentration], thanks to our "precious" auxiliaries . . .);
> 3. because there is no room for error regarding its posology for chemoprophylaxis and thus spares brains that should not be overloaded from all [need for] calculation.[32]

Six months after the accidents of Nkoltang, more than a year before those of Yokadouma, the danger of using Lomidine in powder form was well known and clearly understood: "The preparation of the solution gives so many opportunities for contamination that I wonder how it is that there are not more 'hiccups.' It must be that the backsides of our clients have a greater natural resistance to infection." Thus, the question that arose was: Why were accidents not more frequent and more serious? "Our brothers of color have a great hold on life and a very high natural resistance to telluric germs," Ziegler suggested. Even when following the instructions as rigorously as possible, he explained:

> The risks of contamination are huge: preparation of the solution in poorly sterilized containers, dust falling into the solution (do not forget we always work outside, half protected from the wind by dirty mats), filling of syringes by drawing from the solution with a contaminated nozzle, etc., etc. The first time I saw this, I was terrified. Since then, I have become more philosophical, yet I still often tremble and there is no reason that the "hiccups" that happened to MAINETTE [should] not happen to me some unlucky day.[33]

Ziegler's unlucky day would come (see chapter 10). In the meantime, he had ideas for fixing the problem: to use Lomidine prepared by Spécia as a sterile solution and packaged in very high-volume flasks (500 cubic centimeters) fitted with a special "distributor" device to prevent contamination of the solution while filling syringes, allowing for serial injections. A sketch of his vision of the ideal flask was included with his letter: the low-volume flasks already on the market were poorly suited to the rhythm of large-scale campaigns. Ziegler's letter made the rounds of Spécia's departments, but the firm in the end did not follow up on the young doctor's proposal: his imagined flask was described as a "very costly 'monster.'"[34]

More accidents took place in 1953. The news reached Spécia, which accelerated the development of high-volume flasks. After Nkoltang and in the face of new accidents in the Haute-Sangha region (in Nola, the city across the border from Yokadouma), AEF announced it would in future order only the solution. Cameroon, however, in an order dated March 19, 1954, remained loyal to the powder, which it purchased in bulk in 250–gram boxes. In the delivery of this order, perhaps, was the box Ansellem would use in Gribi in November. At Spécia, news of that accident would elicit anger: "It is against our repeated advice to use solution that Cameroon has persisted in asking for powder for reasons of cost."[35] Seen from the factories of Saint-Fons, the catastrophe of Yokadouma happened in slow motion.

The Accident Did Not Happen

The incident at Yokadouma led to a sudden drop in the Lomidinization statistics in Cameroon in a context of growing tension. With the riots of May 1955, the country descended into violence; protesters were shot by the army right in front of the head office of the public health service and the SHMP. In July 1955, the UPC was banned.

On July 7, 1956, the state prosecutor for Yaoundé's Court of Appeal, identified only as Laborde, sent the high commissioner of the French Republic in Cameroon, Pierre Messmer, his confidential opinion on the "affair of the deaths of Yokadouma."[36] Eighteen months had gone by since the last deaths; the definitive toll was 30 deaths and 320 "serious accidents." The question was whether there should be any further legal action: the state prosecutor was empowered, in the name of the "public prosecutor," to bring the case before the court. In four pages, the prosecutor summed up the judicial inquiry. His conclusions deliver a last, definitive blow to the image of a functional colonial medical and administrative machine.

The prosecutor's conclusions confirmed the inquiry's. Thanks to the results of bacteriological testing, the judicial inquiry had validated, with absolute certainty, the scenario of an accident caused by contamination of the Lomidine solution, as well as the negligence of team chief Ansellem.

Yet the prosecutor introduced a series of conflicting elements. The first was disclosed from the outset: the official instructions for the use of Lomidine had not been complied with in Yokadouma. The prosecutor specified: "The solvent should have been lukewarm saline solution (circular 6609 DH, August 12, 1954, from the chief of the SHMP), a practice that was abandoned because it was too costly (report 90/CF, November 24, 1954, from the chief of the SHMP)." In August 1954, probably following the reoccurrence of post-injection incidents, Dr. Cauvin indeed made an adjustment to the Lomidinization technique in a circular addressed to all team chiefs, which specified—this is the point that attracted the judicial inquiry's attention—that the injection had to be prepared with "saline solution." Given the vast scale on which campaigns were running in 1954, the application of this directive would have required the production of saline on a quasi-industrial scale. Cauvin therefore had to explain in his post-accident report that "this method of operation could not be put into practice because it turned out to be much too costly."[37] In sum, the administration, by contravening its own instructions, had put itself in an awkward situation.

This was just the first in a long list of inconsistencies that Laborde laid out to justify his position, which was that charging Ansellem in the criminal court for involuntary harm and manslaughter was indeed an option, "yet this solution, while it might seen appropriate in terms of the law, is not in terms of equity." For the prosecutor, a number of factors had to be added to the equation, tipping it toward an indictment of the administration itself. First of all, the investigation had not been sufficiently thorough, and the affair was referred to the magistrates too late. Moreover, the very organization of Lomidinization by the SHMP was open to criticism: "It seems in addition that the equipment provided to health assistants was insufficient; that Ansellem, a dental technician, had inadequate professional training; that the accident that happened to him using a filter in poor condition could just as well have occurred in the days that followed with the SHMP's supposedly acceptable filter had it deteriorated without him noticing."[38]

In the space of a paragraph, the prosecutor pointed, for the first time in this affair, to problems inherent to the campaign: the equipment, the qualifications of the team chief, and that the safety of the chain as a whole depended on the quality of the filters, which was difficult to check. This, to some extent, called into question the normal, day-to-day functioning of mobile teams. Prosecutor Laborde's reading of the incident thus diverged from the register of "unfortunate accident" and "individual negligence." The problem was no longer a grain of sand in the machine; it was the machine itself: "If Ansellem thus committed a minor personal fault, the service's failings seem much more serious, and this is why I believe that I must, for the sake of equity, request a dismissal in this case."

The prosecutor defended his case for dismissal by considering the health assistant to be a mere cog within a service that disregarded its own precautionary instructions. Yet this judgment was also opportune, in the best interest of the state itself, because the conclusions were embarrassing, and a dismissal had the advantage of discretion:

> The administration will find [a dismissal] to be in its interest by avoiding a public debate, in the course of which the methods of the Service de santé could be criticized.
>
> In addition, the solution of referring Ansellem to the criminal court would

have as a consequence to elicit the constitution of many civil parties on the part of victims and families who were probably already compensated by the administration but who would nevertheless put forward new claims, which would be only platonically satisfied by the conviction of Ansellem for damages, since he appears to be devoid of resources.

I must however specify on this point that about thirty persons have already brought civil actions to the investigation and that they will need to be notified of the dismissal. This being an affair that is likely to lead to political repercussions, given the number of victims and the fact that a service of the Territory could be indicted, I would be grateful if you could please let me know if you approve my point of view.[39]

The archives do not reveal what the High Commission replied to the prosecutor's proposal.

The Accident as Moment of Truth

In proposing this arrangement, the prosecutor's confidential letter paints a bleak, but not really surprising, picture of colonial justice in Cameroon in the late 1950s. The administration had, over the previous year, orchestrated a violent repression of the UPC; its energies were focused on "pacifying" the Bassa country, where militants of the national liberation movement had started going underground. That the affair of Yokadouma was dispatched with a dismissal does not in this context seem shocking. It would have taken more, as a "war without a name" was breaking out, to raise a scandal.

Yet Laborde's line of argument did put forward a new interpretation of the iatrogenic accident: it was the product of the rational organization of the campaigns rather than unpredictable error. Accidents reveal most about norms, not because they transgress them, but rather because they are produced by them. To follow Michel Foucault in this argument, iatrogenic accidents should be ascribed "to the action of medical intervention itself, in its rational foundations."[40] Through the lens of the prosecutor's unofficial request for a dismissal, medical practices in their very normality appear as problematic: for six years, as it implemented Lomidinization, the SHMP had been operating as an organization that was in breach of duty. By drawing attention to this embarrassing situation, where the doctor in chief recommended the use of saline solution and then chose not to use it for "economic reasons," the prosecutor questioned the calculations of cost-efficiency used to justify giving priority to mass medicine over investing in health-care facilities. The hospital in Brazzaville, it was said, cost as much to run as all of the mobile teams of AEF put together.[41] By pointing out a risk that was inherent to these rational calculations, the prosecutor underlined—this was rarely voiced during the colonial period—the irreducible risk of mass medicine, caught up as it was in the contradictions of the ever so modern injunction to crunch the numbers and quantify everything.

The real flaw in the affair was a cold-blooded calculation. Interviewed in 2003, a member of the SHMP still remembered that the incident of Yokadouma was an "idiotic matter of a filter" and an economic choice by the head of the department, which turned out to be dangerous:

> But there were accidents; in Yokadouma, there were, I don't know . . . ninety [*sic*]
> deaths. Simply because a head of the Service de santé had decreed that ampules
> of saline for diluting Lomidine were too expensive, so water had to be filtered, it
> had to be boiled. What was forgotten is that a filter . . . gets shaken up. You move
> it around in a truck, you know the SHMP trucks, that was an adventure. There's
> a filter that cracked and it let [in] some *Bacillus perfringens*, and so we inoculated
> some *perfringens* into the poor fellows. There were, I don't know, eighty deaths.[42]

The accident of Yokadouma also laid bare the impotence of colonial public health. This does not mean one should underestimate the violence of the campaigns or the brutality of the damage: "All we did was carry out the law that made Lomidine compulsory and that brought us death," the canton chiefs put it plainly.[43] But it is important to point out that the accident revealed a mediocre medicine, which could not manage to apply its own rules.

Prosecutor Laborde's analysis, in expressing concern about Ansellem's lack of training, draws attention to the extent to which the grand programs of postwar public health depended on a massive use of subalterns. For doctors seeking explanations for Lomidinization accidents, nurses and health assistants were the main source of the problems. Responding to Nkoltang, Muraz had recommended that Lomidinization campaigns be headed only "by a doctor . . . and not only and exclusively by African nurses." The accident merely revealed the extent of the problem: "Yet once again and about these *exceptional* incidents, arises the question of the inadequacy of the medical personnel posted in the bush of our black Africa."[44] In November 1954, Cauvin came to the same conclusions about the catastrophe of Yokadouma. He called for a reorganization of the map of public health to "prevent health agents from being constantly left to themselves" and to put an end to the recruitment of contract workers (*contractuels*), a "category of personnel . . . very often technically inadequate given that the pay that they are allocated does not match what is asked of them."[45]

The accident of Yokadouma reveals the utterly banal side of colonial medicine: the staff of a mobile team was made up of nurses, porters, and orderlies and, at the supervisory level, health assistants and "African doctors"; the presence of colonial doctors was exceptional. It was lamented in 1954 that only about thirty colonial doctors were posted in Cameroon, down from nearly fifty in the 1930s. The pressures of the Indochina war had added to the chronic difficulties of recruitment; a reliance on subalterns, who were much cheaper, grew in the 1950s. Yet the problem was not with the African doctors trained in Dakar, who were never blamed for any of the accidents. Indeed, the racial division of the work set their status as auxiliaries, and they were restricted to fixed postings in dispensaries; it was said they were not versed in the subtleties and cunning of command. Instead, European contractual doctors and European health assistants were preferably entrusted with the responsibility of heading mobile teams. The French and Belgian colonial medical enterprises were, from the beginning of the twentieth century, also an enterprise of Hungarians, Italians, and Russians; in Cameroon, the first Lomidinization of the focal area of Yokadouma was the work of Dr. Valkevitch.[46] "There were a few civilians who were on contracts, hired by army officers, very badly paid, who were made to do the lowest jobs. . . . You know these were fellows who were a bit . . . fellows who were a bit shady . . . after the war. . . . some guys from Central Europe who had slightly dubious diplomas . . . guys like that. So there were a few contract workers in Cameroon. . . . they were Italian[s], a few Czechs."[47]

Often, the only medical staff on tours were these jacks-of-all-trades of colonial medicine; a few hundred of them were spread out across the empire, such as Ansellem, the main character of the affair of Yokadouma, whose trace in the archives is very hard to find. A witness's account of the affair confirms this picture:

> *The treatment team, was it punished?*
>
> No, it wasn't punished but they got stuck, they shut themselves up in a house. They just managed to make it, you know. . . . The rescue team, we might say, arrived soon enough to prevent them from being lynched. There was a European and some Africans.
>
> *And the European, was he military?*

No. He was a contract worker. For that dirty work, it was always contract workers. The subaltern employees of the Service de santé were not doctors, were not government agents, they were on contract. I think, at the time, they made 30,000 francs per month. They weren't rolling in money, were they?

And where did they come from?

From everywhere; a majority were French. For those I came across, there were some ex-non-coms [noncommissioned officers] who had retired, some nurses, some ex-nurses. From Brittany, generally. There were a few Italians. Oh, there weren't many. For all of Cameroon they were maybe fiftyish. Not even.

And it was these guys who were in the regions.

They didn't have a fixed address. They had their trucks, their army cots, they set out and went from village to village. And they were allowed a guest hut when they were in Yaoundé or in a capital. You know, they weren't pampered.[48]

The catastrophe at Yokadouma shows another picture of the practice of mass medicine—the flip side of the image of colonel-doctors of the colonial corps parading in their spotless uniforms in African capitals. Yokadouma suggests that for any instance of standard medicine, there was very often only the work of an Ansellem, a dental technician turned "health assistant," left to himself and underpaid, in some godforsaken place with his gun, his "boy," his whiskey, his five syringes, his ten needles, and his four nurses.

CHAPTER TEN

The Swan Song of Eradication

In September 1958, Georges Neujean, the Belgian director of the BPITT (the institution that coordinated sleeping sickness control across Africa) presented a paper on the chemotherapy and chemoprophylaxis of sleeping sickness caused by *T. gambiense* at the sixth International Congress of Tropical Medicine in Lisbon. Speaking to sleeping sickness experts, Neujean, the most highly respected Belgian colonial doctor of his time, reviewed the "unprecedented success" and "extraordinary" results of pentamidinization. With rates of the virus in circulation tending toward zero, the disease was becoming impossible to map: "The question is not so much to reduce the endemic but rather to seek to erase it." There were, of course, plenty of problems, as Neujean pointed out: some undisciplined individuals managed to avoid injections; some were not adequately protected by the preventive injection—the duration of its efficacy was not known for sure—while some who carried the parasite were not properly detected and were thus exposed to hidden infections by the injection of pentamidine. Nevertheless, Neujean continued, "these considerations cannot make us hesitate to undertake chemoprophylaxis campaigns in endemic regions *as long as we are guaranteed to be able to see them through*—because we knowingly sacrifice individuals in the aim of solving a collective problem."[1]

In just a sentence, Neujean summed up the logic, the absurdity, and the drama of pentamidinization's final years. A series of terrible accidents, coming on top of the drug's intrinsic limitations, had shifted the perspective on preventive pentamidine: by now, it was clear to everyone that the method exposed individuals to significant risk. But for this colonial doctor, who had orchestrated pentamidinization campaigns in Congo, this danger was yet another reason to step up the effort "because we knowingly sacrifice individuals in the aim of solving a collective problem." This sentence—which would be cut from the published version—is worth reading again, because it was not a metaphor. No, what Neujean, a leading expert in tropical medicine and supposedly a man of compassion, who oversaw the Queen Astrid Charity for Native Maternal and Child Welfare in the Belgian Congo,[2] was saying is that not only did the duty of eradication impose the need to bring death to some individuals, but also that these sacrifices would be meaningful only if campaigns were led with the energy required to "see them through." Neujean, no doubt, was alluding to the troubles proliferating across Africa, which were turning injection campaigns into policing operations.

A peculiar narrative—part assessment, part anticipation—was taking shape in the late 1950s. It was articulated in the future perfect tense: Lomidinization will have eradicated sleeping sickness, and colonial medicine will thereby have accomplished its greatest contribution to Africa's future. These things would happen unless "political conditions" intervened and ruined everything, preventing the completion of the enterprise, in which case not only would the disease come back but also those who will have been consciously sacrificed for the good of all will have died for naught, not because of a drug, but because of the selfishness and ungratefulness of Africans.

This success story, attached to a desperate and reactionary meditation on decolonization, was to be pentamidinization's swan song.

The Last Inventory

Sleeping sickness chemoprophylaxis came to a brief climax. While everywhere campaigns were slowing down and new infections becoming exceedingly rare, the scientific celebration of the method could count on the statistical achievements of more than ten years of mass campaigns on an international scale.

In August 1958, Commander-Doctor Jean Demarchi, the director of the Institut Pasteur of AEF in Brazzaville, presented the most comprehensive study to date on the implementation of chemoprophylaxis at a meeting of the CSIRT (Comité scientifique international pour les recherches sur la trypanosomiase; International Scientific Council for Trypanosomiasis Research and Control) in Brussels.[3] His report compiled summaries requested of the French, Portuguese, Belgian, and British health services. This act of inventorying gave chemoprophylaxis, a posteriori, the coherence of an international eradication program; it also gave retrospective meaning to the public health collaborations among the colonial powers—at the very moment when the emergence of the WHO signaled the end of the ephemeral era of inter-imperial health.

The statistics showed a marked decline in activity since the apex of the campaigns circa 1954. In Cameroon, the shock of the accident of Yokadouma had led to an interruption of campaigns across most of the territory. Lomidinization then was used parsimoniously only in the very north, far from the political unrest in the south, or in "useful" regions such as Mungo, where a significant workforce was employed by banana plantations. In Njombé, two deaths by syncope occurred in August 1957. Although these accidents did not overly disconcert doctors, who attributed them to alcohol consumption despite the early hour of the injection sessions, they did precipitate the end of Lomidinization in Cameroon.[4] In AOF, Lomidinization was also limited to a few "very restricted regions, cantons or even villages" and to the employees of a few plantations;[5] in Côte d'Ivoire, a nurses strike prevented the execution of the last scheduled campaign. There were nowhere near the hundreds of thousands of injections administered annually only a few years before: in the reports sent to Demarchi, there was no attempt to even tally the totals. In AEF, the number of injections had halved since the accidents of 1952–53. In the Belgian Congo, the campaigns were maintained, but without conviction. Official reports did not bother giving more than the bare figures, or else they "cut-and-pasted," restating word for word the self-satisfied declarations of prior reports—such was the boredom of success.[6] Only Angola and Portuguese Guinea stepped up the cadence of campaigns, perhaps because the political situation in Portuguese Africa was not a source of worry for the colonial administration.

This dip in statistics was presented as a tactical adjustment: in the future, sleeping sickness control would consist of treating the handful of cases showing up in dispensaries. Health services could now focus on other public health issues: in the late 1950s, the mobile teams broadened their targets to include additional "social endemics." French-style mass medicine became a model, which even had its followers in British Africa. From 1956, leprosy, tuberculosis, onchocerciasis, and gonorrhea were targeted by mobile campaigns aiming to reduce the virus reservoir with new drugs and vaccines. The methods of the injection campaigns were transferred to other programs. In 1955, for example, an international program was launched to eradicate yaws (a disabling skin disease similar to syphilis, caused by a treponema) with intramuscular injections of PAM penicillin,[7] which were administered in endemic zones to the entire population. A single injection could cure patients and stop transmission. An injection in the buttocks—it was the same medical gesture, and the experience of Lomidinization could be put to good use. Nurse-injectors were recycled, and colonial experts reinvented themselves. Colonel-Doctor Lotte, the great Lomidinizer of AEF, for example, represented France at the yaws conference organized under the auspices of the WHO in Enugu, Nigeria,[8] while Raymond Beaudiment, the former head of campaigns in Cameroon, was cited, somewhat ironically, as an expert on accidents linked to intramuscular injections.[9]

Now that the sleeping sickness crisis had been defused, the ending of pentamidinization was presented as a strategic decision dictated by both public health priorities and political difficulties.

A Monument to the Colonial Past

The swan song of pentamidinization also announced the end of the interimperial form of collaboration initiated by the BPITT in Léopoldville. Even before independence, the launching of malaria and yaws eradication programs, as well as the establishment in Brazzaville of the African headquarters of the WHO, ushered in the era of international public health in Africa. This handover was experienced with some bitterness by Belgian and French doctors, who worried about interference from the WHO and briefly attempted to make the strategic move of turning the BPITT into an institution with a broader mandate of responsibility for health issues in Africa.[10] With the exception of the Portuguese colonies, independence was granted to the territories that had been touched by Lomidinization in the years between 1957–58 (for Ghana and French Guinea) and 1962 (Rwanda and Burundi), with the majority, from Cameroon to the Belgian Congo, gaining independence in 1960. The parenthesis of "social colonialism" was closed.

Medicine's institutional landscape was profoundly transformed: in the space of a few months, the joint creation by French colonial doctors and governments of the new African states of two new international organizations, the OCCGE and the OCEAC, and of the Instituts Pasteur of Yaoundé and Bangui, gave a future to French medicine in Africa.[11] From Yaoundé to Bobo-Dioulasso, commemorations of the heroes of colonial medicine, from Muraz to Jamot, multiplied; the colonial medical enterprise could now be reinterpreted as the early incarnation of a Franco-African relationship that was being redefined, post-independence, as one of friendship and technical assistance. The success of the fight against sleeping sickness became both a memorial and a blueprint for the future.[12] In the former colonies, paths diverged: in what had been French Africa, the number of doctors from the colonial corps *increased* after independence,[13] while in Léopoldville during the panic of the July 1960 riots, the majority of the Belgian doctors fled the country.

The writing of pentamidinization's final assessment took place in this uncertain climate of both political vacuum and institutional upheaval. It functioned as an endorsement, to which was added the weight of the WHO's new authority—a prestigious UN institution, unencumbered by the label of colonialism. In a special issue of the WHO's *Bulletin*, a section on the method was based on the proceedings of a 1962 expert meeting in Geneva.[14] In the company of Marcel Vaucel and Georges Neujean, who published a sanitized version of the report he had presented in Lisbon in 1958, Jean Schneider, a professor of tropical disease at the Faculté de médecine in Paris, praised pentamidine chemoprophylaxis as a "true revolution" instigated by Professor Launoy. The millions of injections were lauded; no doubts were raised. There was even self-congratulation in having demonstrated, at long last, the drug's lasting retention by the organism. An experiment conducted for Spécia by Launoy and Jonchère (a retired colonial doctor now at the Parisian firm) was exhumed to show, using a radioactive tracer, that pentamidine was stored "in the viscera" and that, by its "slow dis-impregnation," the active substance was made available in the human organism over an extended period of time. (These conclusions would be completely invalidated by pharmacodynamic studies conducted in the 1980s.) But Schneider enthusiastically concluded that modern science had provided a posteriori proof for the practice, which "added another argument, if that was even necessary, in favor of the extension and generalization of this method to all territories where endemic sleeping sickness reigns";[15] eradication, the "ultimate goal," would soon be achieved. Schneider seemed to be speaking in both the future and past tenses: as he wrote this call to general mobilization, Lomidinization campaigns had been ceased in nearly all of Africa.

From the BPITT to the WHO, from reports to articles, from conferences to committees, edifying stories about vanquished epidemic foci and heedless Africans circulated. As is often the case, in the acts of copying and translation, such statements gained stability and authority—in other words, common sense was manufactured. This is what happened with the interpretation of deaths following injection as due to the "pusillanimity" or "emotiveness" of some ethnic groups, which made its way into every overview of the topic, including a Portuguese publication dated as late as 1971.[16] This was also the case for explanations of the gangrene epidemics. Demarchi in his 1958 report explained, without compunction, that a "very thorough judicial investigation" had shown that the gangrenes of Nkoltang were caused by people's application of a "plaster [made from] wet excrement, mud and mashed banana, commonly used in the region as an anti-inflammatory."[17] And Schneider explained to the WHO that the investigation had revealed that "the victims were the ones responsible, having applied, at the site of injection, a particularly septic plaster (mixtures of mud, excrement and mashed banana)."[18] Both of these were word-for-word restatements, years after the accidents, of the fables of Richet and Muraz, who had deliberately contradicted the actual reports of the investigations. It might be added that Jean Schneider worked as a scientific advisor to Spécia; apparently, obscenity pays.[19]

Although the method was being celebrated one last time, reality nonetheless had to be acknowledged: campaigns were becoming impossible, Africans were fleeing the injections, and in some places the epidemic was resurgent. "The fire smolders under the ashes," reported Demarchi in 1958 with reference to AEF. In the field, few doctors still used the method without apprehension: they feared accidents as much as popular defiance in regions that had been Lomidinized up to "12 or 13 times."[20] "Psychological factors" were evoked with alarm; they would ruin everything.[21] A general discrediting of the method was on the horizon; it had, essentially, been initiated by its subjects; independence only provided a convenient explanation for abandoning the method. In 1962 in Congo, the people of the "old lands of sleep[ing sickness]" refused Lomidinization.[22]

The experts' declarations of faith thus went hand in hand with a warning: the failure of eradication, if it were to happen, would have to be blamed on politics. In August 1958, after listening to Demarchi, the experts at the Brussels meeting solemnly issued a set of recommendations. Their credo reaffirmed, louder than ever, the "excellent results" of preventive pentamidine, even if its mysterious mode of action, they admitted, needed further research: the only obstacles were "of an administrative, social and economic nature."[23] Preventive pentamidine worked—how and for how long, no one knew—but it worked, and the only danger was the emerging disorder, declared the specialists. "The root of the medical problem [had] become political," Neujean explained to the WHO in 1963. The technique being infallible, and the population ungrateful or ignorant, the coming failure would be a confirmation of the starting premise.

CHAPTER ELEVEN

How the Drug Became Useless and Dangerous

Celebrated yet abandoned in practice by the end of colonial rule, pentamidinization's very principle was thrown into question in the 1960s. A new generation of doctors and researchers, some African, demonstrated that pentamidine had no preventive effects per se, and they completely reinterpreted how the drug had curbed the epidemics of the 1940s. It was discovered—to many people's displeasure—that pentamidinization had "worked" by treating, unintentionally and imperfectly, a vast reservoir of infected individuals who were mistakenly identified as healthy. Thus, pentamidinization had acted not by preventing new infections in healthy individuals, but rather by treating, unknowingly and on a massive scale, parasite carriers who were not detected in the course of screening. In this new world, where colonialism no longer reigned, the whole history of pentamidine needed to be rewritten; it became an embarrassing, almost incomprehensible, episode in the history of tropical medicine.

The Key to the Mystery

How was the mystery of the drug's prodigious yet erratic effects solved? A fresh clue had made its way into experts' discussions. In the early 1960s, a new testing technique based on so-called B2M (blood proteins of the immunoglobulin family) turned the diagnosis of the disease on its head. The technique made it possible to identify probable trypanosome carriers by measuring their levels of B2M; abnormally high levels are an indicator of immunological reaction to the parasites. (This principle—detecting infections indirectly via their immunological traces in the organism—is commonplace in current diagnostic methods.)

This new testing device was much trickier to use in the field than the painstaking search by microscope for parasites wriggling in a drop of blood.[1] Yet its sensitivity was much greater, and the test could thus reveal the hidden part of the iceberg: the huge number of parasite carriers who, until then, were wrongly considered to be healthy. It became clear that microscopic screening was, on its own, ineffective; there was no need to invoke the indiscipline of patients or nurses' lack of vigilance. The blood tests performed to prepare for Lomidinization missed a large number of positives, notably in cases of recent infection.

In this context, the doubts that had cropped up in the scientific literature of the 1950s made their way to the crux of the debate. In the field of tropical medicine, a controversy broke out. Among French experts, the confrontation took place on the stage of the first technical conference of the OCEAC, which met in Yaoundé in early December 1965. About fifty delegates were gathered: French military doctors, former colonials turned technical assistants, American observers, and representatives of the region's governments, of the WHO, and of pharmaceutical firms, including Spécia. The entire Franco-African public health scene was in Yaoundé for what would become, until the 1980s, a regular meeting. Dr. Aujoulat, who was in charge of cooperation at the Ministère de la santé in Paris, represented France; Dr. Vaucel was sent by the Institut Pasteur of Paris; Dr. Labusquière, who had experimented with Lomidine on himself in 1945 as a doctor in chief in Ayos, Cameroon, was now the general secretary of the OCEAC; and Dr. Ziegler, who had made a name for himself in 1948 with a brilliant MD thesis on Lomidine, represented the Service des grandes endémies (Service for Major Endemic Diseases), where he was now pursuing his career.

A session was devoted to trypanosomiasis, which was essentially a theoretical issue now that "the indices are all expressed as zero point zero something" and preventive Lomidine was generally no longer in use.[2] Jean Dutertre, who was working for the OCEAC in Yaoundé, nonetheless undertook to provide an overview of chemoprophylaxis, "whose use kindled such great hope and had put the term eradication back on the agenda."

"The prophylactic activity of Lomidine poses a few problems," he began. Besides the usual question regarding its biological action—that is, "should we accept that [Lomidine] is present, in circulation, over a period of six months, at a high enough concentration to prevent infestation?"—an alternative hypothesis for its effects was emerging. The supposition was that Lomidinization was not truly prophylaxis, but rather an indiscriminate treatment, and the "prophylactic" action was, in fact, the effect of a reduction in the virus reservoir at the scale of a population. Accordingly, Lomidinization had acted "only by eliminating circulating trypanosomes" in a large number of subjects who were infected yet identified as healthy by screening tests that were *ineffectual*, as proven by the method of B2M.

It was a minor bombshell: the new testing method indeed made visible a set of healthy carriers who, until then, had been undetected and had been subjected to "preventive" (scare quotes were now mandatory) Lomidinization. Taking this element into account, which was rather unsettling for the veterans of *la trypano*, brought the fundamental principle of chemoprophylaxis crashing down:

> This would mean that the recurrence of infestation was prevented not by the protection of contacts, but by the momentary sterilization of the endemic focus. This sterilization would seem to mask foci rather than eliminating them, if it is true that the bipolar principle of prophylaxis:
>
> 1. detection and elimination of virus carriers
> 2. protection of the uninfected population
>
> in reality consisted of:
>
> 1. detection and elimination of some virus carriers
> 2. momentary sterilization of a greater number of virus carriers.[3]

This new conception of Lomidinization amounted to seeing it as "a treatment in disguise, most often an insufficient one, but which palliates incomplete screening." This was not just a theoretical problem. It was possible that preventive Lomidine was the cause of a resurgence in atypical, difficult-to-treat forms of infection, a result of single administrations of insufficient doses of the drug. In conclusion, not only was there "no hope for eradication by this method, [which has been shown] therefore [to be] exclusively palliative," but the question of its risks was also posed: risks for the individual being exposed to a second-rate treatment and—this was the last straw—risks for the collective, which had been exposed to a stubborn virus reservoir created by the drug.

The presentation provoked a spirited discussion—though surely softened by friendly relations—among the experts in the audience. An elegant scientific argument was evoked to support the new theory: the exclusively therapeutic— that is, not preventive—effect of Lomidine on *T. rhodesiense* (the East African trypanosome) provided a demonstration that its prophylactic power was an epidemiological illusion produced by the interruption of transmission at the level of a population. Indeed, it was well known that, unlike *T. gambiense*, *T. rhodesiense* had a reservoir in wild animals, which, obviously, was out of the reach of injection campaigns. As Dutertre joked, "it would be necessary," in order to generate the impression of a preventive effect, "to Lomidinize, in addition to the whole population, every bushbuck in the territory."

Doubts ran through the experts. Could they "contemplate Lomidinization only after immunological testing?" wondered Dutertre. Should they "repudiate the value of preventive Lomidinization in individual cases?" asked the head of the Service des grandes endémies of Cameroon. Could they not "continue Lomidinizing in individual cases?" insisted Labusquière, the secretary general of the OCEAC. Could it really be true that preventive Lomidine did not protect individuals?

Marcel Vaucel, the most senior and illustrious figure in the room, spoke up several times to reaffirm his trust in the technique. "The prophylactic effect of Lomidinization was proven in animals," he pointed out; its efficacy on a collective scale, no matter what the theoretical explanation, was undeniable. Vaucel reiterated: "Some [of its] results have been remarkable, that these might be a result of the elimination of the virus reservoir is [certainly] possible, yet this remains the most advisable operation when there is a threat." Still, when it came to the case of the individual, rather than that of an endemic focus to be brought under control, Vaucel felt the need to discuss Lomidine's risk-benefit ratio: "It is preferable not to Lomidinize individuals who cannot be medically monitored. It is preferable to be diagnosed as infected and treated, rather than to be Lomidinized and then become unknowingly infected. While it is good in mass practice, it is not so great in individual practice."[4]

This calculus was both novel and cautious. Lomidine remained advisable for the "mass," which benefited from the drastic drop in transmission rates that followed from blindly treating healthy carriers. Yet it had become useless in "individual practice," for example, in "soldiers going for survival training in the bush." Even for migrant workers, who were customarily Lomidinized either when they passed through border posts or when they were recruited at work sites, preventive injections were now debatable, especially if the migrants were under regular medical monitoring and so could be treated if they became infected. Thus, the distinction between the individual and the mass, which historically had been anchored in the European–African racial distinction, was reinterpreted in terms of access to medical care. The individual was defined as someone who could be followed in a dispensary. The rest were collective beings, epidemic focuses to be Lomidinized.

Not everyone defended this risk-benefit calculus. Standing by his convictions, Jacques Pierre Ziegler said that "he had had the opportunity to Lomidinize Chadian workers on their way to Gabon, and that he [in any case] would Lomidinize them." Certainly, the credibility of individual prophylaxis had been considerably weakened: for healthy individuals, unless they were part of an endemic area to be quelled, Lomidine was no longer of any value. Certainly, the retrospective reinterpretation of how Lomidinization had worked now tipped a decade of theory into the realm of illusion and error: the only so-called prophylaxis had been the massive and clumsy treatment of an unsuspected virus reservoir. Certainly, the theories that had explained the feats of the miracle drug, a drug that sterilized flies and protected villages for years at a time, now, in retrospect, verged on the ridiculous. And yet, the new theory also viewed Lomidinization from a population-level perspective, which remained the hard core of sleeping sickness control. Colonial doctors were able, in a way, to land on their feet: they had always seen Lomidine as a drug for the masses rather than as an individual prophylactic. This time, they had proof of it.

A Final Incident

One more incident would put the final nail in the coffin of the method's credibility. The fatal blow landed *during* the OCEAC conference of 1965, a few thousand kilometers from Yaoundé in southern Chad. Coincidentally, it threw into relief the lack at the conference of any discussion of side effects and accidents.

On Monday, December 6, 1965, a team from Chad's Service des grandes endémies was conducting a Lomidinization campaign in the village of Goro in the area of Fort Archambault (now Sahr). The medical workers Lomidinized the village and then continued the campaign. Two days later, the team found out there had been two fatalities in Goro. Over the next days, the tragic scenarios of Nkoltang and Yokadouma were replayed with relentless accuracy; the final toll reached fourteen deaths. The official summary followed the script of the reports written about the two previous catastrophes, complete with a detailed chronology and little games of investigative deduction—the Lomidinization accident had become a literary genre.[5] The report thus described the organization of the emergency response, the transport of victims to the hospital, the cases of gas gangrene, the autopsies, and finally, the identification of *Clostridium perfringens* at the Brazzaville Institut Pasteur. There was a detailed account of the "careful investigation," with the usual distribution of roles: Lomidine as blameless, nurses' "dubious" testimonies, and the technical error of a subaltern: "It seems that the nurse in charge of preparing [an antiseptic solution] delegated it to an orderly, who . . . made a mistake."[6]

The account gives an impression of déjà vu. Although it did not mention the accidents of Yokadouma or Nkoltang, it reiterated the confident recommendations of previous reports: the method was not to be blamed, and the fault "of a nurse . . . can be considered to be responsible for the death[s] of 14 persons and of the mutilation of 5 more." In future, all would go well: as long as campaigns were supervised by a doctor or by "a competent and conscientious technical agent . . . no serious accident should arise."

The conclusions are astounding. The accident of Chad even raised a tragic paradox to a new level of absurdity: *no one* had been found infected in the focal area by the previous medical screening, and it was "*as a precautionary measure* [that it had been] decided to maintain Lomidinization" (emphasis added). At the time of the accident, the campaign's supervisor was at the OCEAC conference where, fittingly, the value and safety of Lomidinization were being thrown into question: that supervisor was Jacques Pierre Ziegler. He was fervently reaffirming his "trust"—against the majority opinion among his colleagues—in a method that had launched his career and that, at that very moment and under his direct responsibility, was adding fourteen fatalities to the body count of its "operational incidents."

The situation seems particularly ironic because Ziegler—who, in his 1953 correspondence with Spécia, had expressed fear that someday, in the course of Lomidinizing, he might have his "unlucky day"—took it upon himself to give an account of the Chad accident at the OCEAC's technical conference in 1967. One delegate commented that cases of similar accidents had been known for more than a decade. Another noted: "possibly, we cannot assign any fault," given that boiling was known to have little effect on gangrene spores. The chairman closed the session by stating with satisfaction that they had "spent a whole half-day saying new things about sleeping sickness."[7]

The accident of Goro in late 1965 testified yet again to the constitutive amnesia and mediocrity of the apparatus for evaluating public health. The context had changed since the late 1950s: to justify Lomidinization, one could no longer invoke a public health emergency or some collective imperative; it had also become tricky to invoke the interests of the individual per se (the "life insurance of Lomidine" of which health propaganda had spoken). Under these new conditions, deliberations around the accident rendered explicit that which was still solid but had previously stayed under the surface as a last-resort justification for Lomidinization: a combination of faith and stupidity. A method that doctors considered to be "dangerous for the individual" had been implemented "by precaution"! The deaths at Goro, Gribi, and Nkoltang were certainly unfortunate, but not hugely problematic: the victims had, in a way, died to save their race. Indeed, Neujean had said so explicitly in 1958. To echo a more general suggestion made by Jean-Pierre Dozon,[8] this is a case where preventive medicine draws attention rather blatantly to the element of superstition that it always mobilizes, without which one cannot understand all that colonial medicine has achieved. I am tempted to describe the Lomidinization recommended by Ziegler in late 1965, which was based on no other reason than serving "as a precautionary measure" and "for trust in the method," as the manifestation of a strange sacrificial ritual, orchestrated by the decidedly incorrigible men of action of the mobile teams. It was literally a matter, to use the expression of a colonial doctor, of "conjuring a plague."[9]

By 1965, the mystique of eradication had been extended to other diseases—notably with the launch of the smallpox eradication program, which recruited Ziegler to conduct its operations in Zaire. Yet pentamidine prophylaxis did not recover from the tragedy of Goro. Acknowledging the new accident, the two military doctors at the helm of the OCEAC, René Labusquière and Jean Dutertre, undertook in an article published in *Médecine Tropicale* to put the method to rest once and for all.[10] They drew up an inventory of its drawbacks: "it brings about increasingly high levels of absenteeism, which takes away its main value"; "always painful, it can lead, in cases of negligence—and who can ensure that there will never be negligence?—to serious accidents"; and finally, "the truly preventive action of Lomidine" was now in question. The tone was cautious, but the conclusions were authoritative: the debate was closed.

Over the next few months, the method was virtually abandoned in African countries. Only the doctors of Portuguese Guinea, the last to call themselves "colonial," continued pentamidinizing more than ever, in the midst of a war of independence, as if to prevent the end of the colonial world. In 1972, more than a hundred thousand individuals were subjected to injections, every six to nine months, in the zones controlled by the Portuguese army.[11]

The Drug That No Longer Worked

The story ends as it began, with an animal experiment. The last act in the burial of preventive Lomidine happened—giving another ironic twist to the story—in Kinshasa (formerly Léopoldville, the capital of the Belgian Congo, which had become Zaire). Arriving there in 1968, Marc Wéry, a Belgian technical assistant, threw himself into "reviving parasitology at Lovanium," a vast campus built in the late 1950s on a hill on the outskirts of the city, which was deserted by the Belgians soon after independence. He witnessed firsthand the resurgence of the epidemic of sleeping sickness, which notably affected the region of Bas-Congo near Kinshasa. By then, pentamidinization was no longer an option: it had left bitter memories, and it was now futile to count on what was called "discipline." At Lovanium, renamed the Université nationale du Zaïre (National University of Zaire), Wéry collaborated with Professor Donatien Kayembe, who headed the biology laboratory of the university clinics. Kayembe was a member of the first generation of Congolese *médecins agrégés* (doctors of medicine who had passed a qualifying examination for a university position) who had trained in Belgium just after independence. They decided to work together on what was then a "fashionable" topic, as Wéry told me in 2008: pentamidine, which was being "much accused of not doing what was expected of it."[12]

Confused as to the true preventive value of pentamidine, Wéry and Kayembe reproduced experiments conducted thirty years earlier by Van Hoof and his team, who had used guinea pigs. The new protocol was more elaborate, using nearly three hundred rats; the pentamidine was supplied by the Spécia representative in Kinshasa. Notably, Wéry and Kayembe introduced a variable: for each batch of rats, they altered the time interval between the preventive injection and the inoculation of trypanosomes in order to evaluate the duration of protection. Most rats were infected much sooner than expected. The results, published in 1972, were unequivocal: "The protective efficacy of Lomidine present in the organism drops rapidly from 1 week to 1 month after administration."[13]

The last pillar had collapsed. The protection conferred by pentamidine in animals appeared to be very short-lived: after two months, it was nearly nonexistent. Neither Van Hoof, who died in 1948, nor Launoy, who died in 1971 to a chorus of tributes, were around to make an attempt at explaining this discrepancy in results, which had been obtained using protocols similar to the original experiments. Kayembe and Wéry were cautious, admitting that "the mechanism of long-term protection was still beyond them," no doubt in order to avoid saying that, strictly speaking, there was hardly any protection at all. Having shown, in another experiment, that injecting a single dose of Lomidine into infected animals was an ineffective and unpredictable therapy, while multiple injections rapidly led to the development of resistance, they ended their discussion with a question: "Yet how many undiagnosed [people infected with trypanosomiasis], in the very early stages of the disease, . . . did indeed receive this semestral 'preventive' injection of 5 mg/kg in the course of pentamidinization campaigns?"[14]

With this remark, defenders of prophylactic Lomidine lost their last mooring. Donatien Kayembe, who received me in 2007 in his office at the university clinics of the University of Kinshasa, remembered creating with this study—he still had its files—"quite a shockwave." Pentamidine, he explained to me, "was not all that preventive."[15]

Lomidinization had worked inadvertently: it had worked by drastically disrupting transmission within endemic areas through the temporary treatment of the virus reservoir composed of undetected parasite carriers; its efficacy had depended on the mass inoculation of people based on belief in its protective effect, which had been "demonstrated" at the individual level only by the experiments, which lacked rigor even to contemporary observers, on the "volunteers" Moya and Bonkumu. Its contribution to the control of sleeping sickness had initially been extraordinary, yet it had taken place, once the epidemics of the late 1940s were brought under control, at the price of sometimes terrible accidents and the production of atypical clinical forms that were more difficult to treat, and even, according to some, the creation of a "beheaded" (brutally but insufficiently treated) infection that ultimately would act as "a factor favorable to epidemics."[16] In the early 1970s, these were the reasons that preventive Lomidinization exited from official recommendations and medical manuals, advised against everywhere except, it was sometimes specified, in places where it was still "believed in."[17]

Gangrene and Oblivion

The history of preventive pentamidine inspires philosophizing. "We no doubt expected too much," Pierre Richet, a strong proponent of French mass medicine, said in 1974, and "we must drop our illusions."[18] Lomidinization would henceforth be dispatched in just a few words by doctors as well as by historians, in most cases only mentioning its contribution to the final victory of the 1950s; only a few ventured a retrospective rereading of its epidemiological effects. Pharmacodynamic studies provided definitive proof of the nonexistence of pentamidine's long-term retention by the organism. The victory had become cumbersome; the "drug for the masses" was growing more and more unintelligible. In 2003, the twenty-first edition of the bible of tropical medicine, *Manson's Tropical Diseases*, explained in its trypanosomiasis chapter, in a sentence that has the weight of a final verdict: "Chemoprophylaxis is no longer of use because of the poor risk benefit ratio owing to the adverse effects of the drugs in use."[19]

The strange and, in the end, banal trajectory of pentamidine, a drug whose indications were changing at the same time as the political, moral, and racial hierarchies that defined colonialism were collapsing, reveals how things and beings, knowledge and society, are transformed together in history. At the demise of the colonial era, "races" and "populations" had to make space for "individuals," which, only a few years earlier, had been unthinkable for Africa; the drug became "pointless, dangerous, and thus pointlessly dangerous," to cite, again, Labusquière.[20] Meanwhile, Africans like Donatien Kayembe became respected scientists, which was certainly unimaginable in 1942, when Van Hoof was pentamidinizing Moya and Bonkumu.

The colonial biography of pentamidine reveals that the grid of ethical analysis, which has become so commonplace and by which we assess the value of a medical treatment at the scale of an individual—collective benefits coming into play only if they are recognized as adding to individual benefits, as in the case of vaccination—was, for a long time, not thinkable in relation to the racialized body of the African. And this was the case even when—this is a crucial point—such a calculation was taken for granted in the case of the European. The disjunction between these two categories of humanity was enunciated, in all its scandalousness, by the doctors who discreetly exchanged instructions and by the sensational accusations of a Cameroonian deputy in November 1954.

In tracing its biography, the historian must nevertheless come to terms with the obvious fact that pentamidine worked to some extent, but not for the reasons that were invoked at the time. The irony of the story is that colonial doctors were particularly concerned with getting the "African masses" to understand how the drug worked and to adhere to the colonizers' eradication project: "natives of all races [were to be] confronted with scientific truth," Léon Launoy wrote.[21] Summoned by mobile teams, Africans alternated between compliance, especially during the postwar epidemics, and rejection, sometimes en masse, of the sleeping sickness shot. Given the fragility of the "scientific truth" involved, it is difficult not to see a rational element in their distrust of Lomidine, especially given that they welcomed other drugs, such as penicillin, with enthusiasm.

In the panic of campaigns going awry, reason and unreason traded places.

This may be why rumors about the campaigns were so worrying to colonial authorities, as if the irrationality and ignorance of which Africans were being accused might, in fact, be a projection of the doctors' enthusiastic and amnesic foolishness. In January and February 1957, the colonial authorities of Cameroon and Oubangui-Chari thus exchanged anxious letters about a "rumor according to which a European who had come from Cameroon intended to kill children using injections" in the region of Haute-Sangha.[22] An inquiry concluded that the rumor was based on incidents that arose in the course of vaccination in British Cameroon—accusing the British was a classic tactic of French colonialism—and "amplified by troublemakers who spread them in the Center and the South," that is, a trick of the UPC. "It is likely," the high commissioner explained to his counterpart in Bangui, "that this alarmist and unfounded news was propagated in your Territory by a few stupid or malicious people from Cameroon."[23] There was no mention of the accident of Yokadouma, which had happened three years earlier, just a few dozen kilometers from the border of Haute-Sangha.

Patients were randomly assigned to receive [inhalations of] pentamidine or placebo according to a randomization chart. . . .

To preserve study blindness, a nail-biting deterrent (Stop 'n' Grow, The Mentholatum Company, Buffalo, New York) was applied to the mouthpiece of the nebulizer before each treatment to mask the characteristic bitter taste of pentamidine.

S. Montaner et al., "Aerosol Pentamidine for Secondary Prophylaxis of AIDS-Related Pneumocystis Carinii Pneumonia: A Randomized, Placebo-Controlled Study," *Annals of Internal Medicine* 114.11 (1991), 949.

Epilogue

I end this story where it began: in Dagenham, East London, where in 1937 the chemist Arthur Ewins synthesized compound MB 800, later renamed pentamidine. In October 2012, as I was finishing the French edition of this book, I made my first visit to the May & Baker factory that, for decades, had manufactured and marketed pentamidine.

The site's doors opened onto a vast emptiness. All that was left of the factory, which had by then been acquired by Sanofi, was an immense expanse of coarse gravel. Sanofi had not left; it had launched an ambitious "rehabilitation" program it called "Business-East" to breathe new life into the site by creating a "science and business park" for biotechnology companies, with a hotel and supermarket.[1] In late 2012, Business-East was inviting investors and entrepreneurs to take part in the adventure of turning Dagenham into a "mini–Silicon Valley."[2]

I was welcomed by Mark Bass, the land development and partnership leader of Business-East, who was responsible for relations with local residents and former factory workers. Bass, a chemist, worked at May & Baker his whole life, as did his son, also a chemist, who we ran into on our walking tour. He was one of a small group of employees still around; they were given the job of shutting down the site by the end of 2013.

We set out together to see what was left of May & Baker and its archives. Large billboards were attached to the fence surrounding the site, displaying the logo of Business-East and beautiful black-and-white photographs from the factory's archives: women working on a production line, scientists behind their microscopes, rugby teams, and calisthenic sessions. These recalled May & Baker's glorious past in the era of miracle drugs, the British Empire, and the big happy Fordist family. In its busiest years, May & Baker employed more than four thousand people in the industrial city of Dagenham.

In one of the remaining buildings, a ballroom with parquet flooring, listed as a heritage site, held an exhibit that traced decade by decade the factory's life, "The Wall of History." Pentamidine was given a single line in the 1950s: "prescribed," the panel explained, "for the prevention and treatment of pneumonia." On the facing column was a timeline for the decade: the winners of the Football Association Cup, the conquest of Everest, and the coronation of Elizabeth II. More space was given over in May & Baker's institutional memory to other wonder drugs, which were displayed under glass in their original boxes, such as penicillin; Gardenal, a barbiturate; and especially MB 693, a sulfonamide synthesized by Arthur Ewins in 1937, shortly before pentamidine. Marketed as Dagenan, after the city's name, it was known especially by its code name: in the midst of the world war, "compound 693" cured Winston Churchill of a bad case of pneumonia and made its way into the British national heritage.[3]

A visit to the archives did not get me very far. In a prefabricated building, files related to the last drug batches manufactured in 2012 were awaiting shipment to the warehouses of the multinational archiving corporation Iron Mountain. A bit of old stuff was still on the shelves. Another chemist, John Witchell, stayed with me and rummaged around. He took out a few old photo albums and reports from the 1960s. "I can get you excited," John gently poked fun at me while reading from a copy of Arthur Ewins's lab notebooks: "MB 693 . . . MB 742. . . . We're almost there." But nothing on MB 800; the photocopy ended.

Witchell remembered most vividly when pentamidine production was restarted briefly in the late 1980s. "The product was dead at the time," and experienced chemists with the know-how to use old equipment were needed because "not everything was written in the instructions." Witchell was part of the team, as was Mark Bass. While standing on a ladder, he remembered pentamidine, remembered how hard it was to produce a sterile powder, remembered the sealing of flasks, purity testing, and yellow stoppers.

Pentamidine did have a second life. Used in the treatment and prevention of pneumocystis pneumonia (PCP), a serious parasitic infection associated with immunosuppression, pentamidine became in the 1980s a vital drug for patients with AIDS.[4] The exponential progression of the AIDS epidemic led, from 1981, to an explosion in the demand for pentamidine, which had been stocked only in small quantities by Spécia and May & Baker to fulfill (rare) orders from Africa; indeed, the story is that the AIDS epidemic was initially detected by the Centers for Disease Control in Atlanta due to an unexplained increase in early 1981 in the use of pentamidine in the United States.[5] In the face of imminent shortages, May & Baker "resuscitated" the drug.[6] Several companies competed in a scientific and industrial race, arbitrated by the US Food and Drug Administration, to market a form of pentamidine that could be inhaled as an aerosol and thus act directly on the lungs without reaching toxic levels in the rest of the organism. An anticipated additional benefit was the potential for a *preventive* treatment for PCP, which was then the main cause of mortality in patients with AIDS.

Pentamidine has made and lost fortunes. The firm Lyphomed, a small manufacturer of generic drugs, obtained exclusive marketing rights in the United States. Its price, nearly a hundred dollars per flask, made the drug extraordinarily profitable while putting it out of many patients' reach. Activists arranged to obtain contraband pentamidine from Mexico and organized a buyers club to import the powder directly from May & Baker. Patients chained themselves to Lyphomed's gates and participated in the design of community trials of the drug: the "Pentamidine Wars"—the expression was coined by Act Up New York[7]—marked the emergence in the United States of a form of militant mobilization and expertise that ushered medicine into a new era.[8] Meanwhile, at Rhône-Poulenc (which had acquired Spécia and May & Baker), the decision was made to kill the Lomidine trademark and launch a new form of pentamidine, Pentacarinat, in 1989. This new drug was no other than the old English pentamidine isethionate powder, the very drug that had caused terrible accidents in the 1950s, now formulated for aerosol administration. But the price had changed: it was now seventeen times higher! And, as a deputy to the French National Assembly noted, the indication had also changed: "Prophylaxis of [PCP] in patients with AIDS takes up the first seventeen lines of its therapeutic indications. Sleeping sickness features in the eighteenth and last line. The other parasitic diseases have completely disappeared from the leaflet, just like the French colonies have disappeared from atlases."[9] What an apt image: the forgotten Lomidine was "just like" the forgotten French colonial past.

The arbitrary increase in pentamidine's price tag made it, de facto, inaccessible to poor patients, whether they were HIV-positive individuals without insurance in the United States or victims of the resurgence of trypanosomiasis in Africa. The magic of "compassionate capitalism" stepped in: in the United States, Lyphomed proudly launched programs to distribute the medicine to "indigents" on the model of "soup kitchens";[10] Aventis (the former Rhône-Poulenc and future Sanofi), after providing the drug at cost in Africa, announced in May 2001 the launch of a vast drug donation initiative with the WHO, which would cover several molecules used in the treatment of sleeping sickness, including pentamidine. According to the firm's estimates, this donation was worth about $50 million over five years.[11] Giving medicines to the poor—and advertising the fact: this program became Sanofi's philanthropic showcase, the cornerstone of its corporate social responsibility activities. Fifty years after colonial propaganda brochures announced the eradication of sleeping sickness, pentamidine was back on glossy paper.

The resurrection of pentamidine did not save Dagenham, however. The factory had begun to slow down in the early 1990s, as Rhône-Poulenc initiated a series of merger-acquisitions that would make Sanofi one of the world's leading pharmaceutical firms. There was little labor conflict. "There was sadness, yes, but no unrest," remembered Mark Bass. The manufacturing of most chemical compounds and antimicrobial drugs was transferred elsewhere, and the Dagenham facility was reoriented toward products with higher added value for the oncology sector. Looking out at the gravel, in the cold wind and silence, Bass pointed to where buildings had stood: "It's hard to imagine the activity that was on the site, day and night."

From Sanofi's point of view, launching Business-East was not just a way of being socially responsible by staying faithful to the spirit of the place and to the generations that had worked at the M&B factory—even taxi drivers, at the time, knew it by these letters. For the site itself has immense value: Dagenham is on the London Underground's Central Line and only a few miles from the city, whose skyline is visible from the rooftops. In London, the Olympic City, the bare land seems to have greater value than the industrial production of pretty much anything. The factory of Dagenham, the former pride and glory of the British Empire, has become a speculative space; its value is that of the volatile, bright future of London's real estate, of finance, and of biotechnologies. Pentamidine has traveled the same path. The British medicine, a discovery of imperial science and the mass medicine technology of postwar welfare states, has become a post-Fordist substance: a globalized pharmaceutical product, its prices fluctuating with investors' speculation, accessible in Africa only thanks to the sleek generosity of a public-private partnership.

"Be part of our community," invites a blue billboard. The slogan of Business-East resonates ironically with the colonial history of pentamidine, a drug that protected communities, but not individuals. "Be part of something amazing," another sign calls out. Sanofi chose the right term. It *is* amazing, magical even, to watch Business-East being presented as a job creation and urban revitalization initiative—after its promoter razed a factory and, over the space of twenty years, let go of thousands of employees. It is just as amazing, even magical, to watch pentamidine return to publicity brochures, a symbol of the altruism of a pharmaceutical firm determined to make it accessible to all, when its *inaccessibility* was orchestrated by the drastic price increase justified by a "research effort" that was conducted in the 1930s with money from British health insurance.

There's a slightly pungent odor—of acid or sulfur. Mark Bass explains, showing me some backhoes at work behind big white tarps, that the ground below the factory floor has been excavated to a depth of several meters, detoxified by washing and rinsing, and then put back. Listening to him, I wonder if historians can do the same: extract the past, rid it of its toxicity, and put it back.

Acknowledgments

On November 12, 2014, the French National Academy of Medicine blacklisted this book. A few weeks after publication of the French edition, it issued a press release to condemn my "instrumentalization of history."[1] "The academy . . . cannot allow denigration of the memory of these men who chose, most often in the name of a humanitarian ideal, to exile themselves thousands of kilometers from their home, and who braved fevers and epidemics, at the peril of their life, to care and to make medical progress."[2] It was time, the academicians wrote, "to reestablish the scientific truth" about Lomidine.

There was something fascinating about their intervention: it gave me the rare pleasure, as a historian, of coming across something that seemed to arrive straight from the past, almost intact, as if untouched by the passage of time. The academicians' explanations were apparently based on an exclusively French scientific literature on Lomidine's benefit-risk ratio dating back to the 1950s; their corporatist defense of colonial doctors seemed to have been written at that time too. More sadly, it was also a reminder that a large segment of the French intellectual and political elites was still incapable in the twenty-first century of articulating anything reasonable about the colonial past. But the most spectacular aspect was the confidence and serenity with which they reasserted that European-style medicine was one of the "positive effects" of colonization and that the "incidents" that occurred "regularly" during campaigns should be counted as such—as mere incidents, as lives lost for a greater good. They reenacted an emotional blackmail familiar to historians of French decolonization: critics of colonialism have to stop because they are hurting the

[1] http://www.academie-medecine.fr/communique-de-presse-un-vaccin-dangereux-a-t-il-ete-administre-a-des-africains-par-les-medecins-coloniaux-francais-entre-1948-et-1960-a-t-on-deli berement-cache-un-scandale-pharmaceutique-au/, accessed September 2, 2016.

[2] "L'académie . . . ne saurait laisser ainsi dénigrer la mémoire de ces hommes qui choisirent, le plus souvent par idéal humanitaire, de s'exiler à des milliers de kilomètres de chez eux, et qui bravèrent les fièvres et les épidémies, souvent au péril de leur vie, pour soigner et faire progresser la médecine."

hearts of well-intentioned humanitarians, who could in turn stop loving and caring for Africans. The old white male French doctors who wrote the press release had obviously not read my book; they had only heard about it in the press, and they apparently thought there was nothing to be learned from it about colonial medicine, Lomidine, or Africa. That arrogant form of epistemic authority—a specific, scientific form of stupidity that Gustave Flaubert named *bêtise*—is exactly what I try to analyze in this book. Given that unhoped-for demonstration of the enduring empire of medical bêtise, I might have been tempted to begin these acknowledgments by thanking the academicians, but their intervention—exactly sixty years after the injection campaign that killed thirty-two people in Gribi on November 12, 1954—too closely resembled an obscene anniversary.

Starting from the beginning, I would like to thank Anne Marie Moulin. She has supervised this work from the very first days, and I am indebted enormously to her unique expertise and enthusiasm. I also had the chance to be guided from the start by Fred Eboko, who is an exceptional mentor and friend.

I thank Vincent Bonnecase, Sophie Vasset, Aïssatou Mbodj-Pouye, Céline Lefève, and Vinh-Kim Nguyen, who have been friendly readers, writing coaches, and expert advisors on various versions of the manuscript. The comments of Jean-Pierre Dozon, Stéphane Van Damme, Dominique Pestre, Bertrand Taithe, and Megan Vaughan on what was then a part of my PhD thesis were very useful; they may recognize their inspirations and reflections in the text. My discussions on injections during the colonial period with Richard Njouom, Régis Pouillot, and François Simon led me to the pentamidine track, where I crossed the path of Jacques Pépin, who generously shared his insights and archives about the drug and the campaigns. I also thank the historians/biographers of drugs for helping me to frame that strange biography, especially Christian Bonah, Anne Rasmussen, Jean-Paul Gaudillière, Maurice Cassier, Jeremy Greene, Deborah Neill, and Laurence Monnais. This work has been nurtured by long-term conversations on medicine, colonial history, and/or Africa with Wenzel Geissler, Ann Kelly, John Manton, Tamara Giles-Vernick, Noémi Tousignant, René Gerrets, Ashley Ouvrier, Fanny Chabrol, Alice Desclaux, Peter Redfield, Frédéric Keck, Thomas Fouquet, Richard Banégas, Xavier Audrain, Alix Héricord, Hélène Thiollet, Caroline Izambert, Odile Goerg, Luc Berlivet, Olivier Doron, Jean-Paul Lallemand, William Schneider, Charles Becker, Jorge Varanda, Kris Peterson, Gabrielle Hecht, Elizabeth Hull, Tara Diener, Pierre-Marie David, and Nancy Hunt. I thank them for their remarks and encouragement.

I am grateful to the organizers and participants of the seminars where I presented the sad and bizarre history of Lomidine. Mark Harrison gave me the first opportunity to speak about it at the Wellcome Unit for the History of Medicine in Oxford in 2006. I then had the chance to present this work at Indiana University, thanks to William Schneider; at the University of Michigan, thanks to Gabrielle Hecht and Nancy Hunt; at the University of Strasbourg, thanks to Christian Bonah and Anne Rasmussen; at the EHESS and CERMES 3, thanks to Maurice Cassier and Jean-Paul Gaudillière; at the Association française d'ethnologie et d'anthropologie, thanks to Fred Le Marcis and Charlotte Brives; at the CEMAf Aix, thanks to Sandrine Musso; at the WHO in Geneva, thanks to Sanjoy Battacharya; at the University of Montreal, thanks to Laurence Monnais; at the Histories of Health Care in Africa conference in Basel, thanks to Lukas Meier; and at the American Association for the History of Medicine, thanks to Mary Webel and Deborah Neill.

Finishing with the end, I thank Paule Constant and Auguste Bourgeade, who have been extraordinary readers of this text, and Philippe Pignarre, who welcomed it at La Découverte. Vinh-Kim Nguyen, Tamara Giles-Vernick, and Nancy Hunt advised generously about its English translation. I thank Jeremy Greene, whose legendary enthusiasm pushed the book toward the English-speaking world, and Jackie Wehmueller, who gave it the extraordinary chance to be published by Johns Hopkins University Press. I also thank Merryl Sloane for her careful editing of the manuscript. And an immense *merci* to Noémi Tousignant, longtime friend and source of inspiration, who transformed herself into a wonderful translator—an expert with words and on African medical histories.

I would like to express my gratitude to the researchers and archivists who guided my investigation, especially Stéphane Kraxner at the Pasteur Institute; Aline Pueyo and Jean-Marie Milleliri at the Pharo archives; and Jean-Paul Bado, Pierre Dandoy, Michel Thomet, and Olivier de Boisboissel. For the images from the archives of the Institute of Tropical Medicine in Antwerp, I am grateful to Dirk Schoonbaert, Jean-Pierre Wenseleers, and Pr. Bruno Gryseels. Marinette Lugagne, Alice and Thierry Botétémé, and Daniel Claude and Elise Wang Sonné generously shared family photographies and stories with me. I am greatly indebted to the people I interviewed, who are too many to name here, for sharing their memories of colonial medicine, of Cameroon, of Africa, and of the drug that was called Lomidine.

My research has benefited from exceptionally favorable conditions thanks to the support of the Institut universitaire de France, the Agence nationale de la recherche sur le sida (project 1299), the AMADES association, the Maison française d'Oxford, and the Institut de recherches pour le développement (IRD). The support of the IRD enabled me, with the help of Roland Waast, to begin my fieldwork in Cameroon. I found an ideal environment in Paris at the SPHERE and CEMAf laboratories, and I would like to thank their directors Pierre Boilley, Karine Chemla, David Rabouin, and Pascal Crozet, as well as Virginie Maouchi. The translation of the book benefited from the support of the Institut universitaire de France.

Following the story of pentamidine led me to many places from Liverpool to Kinshasa, where I was welcomed and guided by wonderful hosts. I especially want to thank in Yaoundé the Centre Pasteur du Cameroun and its successive directors Jocelyn Thonnon, Jocelyne Rocourt, and Dominique Baudon; the Fondation Paul Ango Ela and its director Kalliopi Ango Ela; the IRD-Yaoundé and its *représentants* François Rivière and Bruno Bordage; Joseph Owona Ntsama, a partner in my research from the beginning; and my colleagues and friends Jean-Pierre Ymele, Sébastien Pion, Michel Boussinesq, Valentin Angoni, Jean Lucien Ewangue, Yves Eyaa, and the very much missed Jean Meno. In Kinshasa, I thank Jacob Sabakinu and Léon Tsambu for their help; in London, Kim Chakanetsa, Romain Denis, and Ninon Fandre; and in Dakar, the whole Zone A team.

And beyond words, I thank my family and friends. I am happy to offer Géraldine and Aimé a book that is about shots that hurt and bulldozers that do not succeed at destroying everything.

Needless to say, I am solely responsible for the content of the book. The bêtises and the mistakes are all mine.

Abbreviations and Acronyms

AA	Archives africaines (African Archives), Brussels
AEF	Afrique équatoriale française (French Equatorial Africa)
AIDS	acquired immune deficiency syndrome
AIPDak	Archives de l'Institut Pasteur de Dakar (Archives of the Pasteur Institute of Dakar)
ANY	Archives nationales du Cameroun (National Archives of Cameroon), Yaoundé
AOF	Afrique occidentale française (French West Africa)
Arch. CSE	Archives de la congrégation des Pères du Saint-Esprit (Archives of the Holy Ghost Fathers Congregation), Chevilly-Larue
Arch. Spécia	Archives Spécia, Sanofi, Société d'archivage moderne (Society for Modern Archiving), Besançon
ATCAM	Assemblée territoriale du Cameroun (Territorial Assembly of Cameroon)
Bib. IMTA	Bibliothèque de Institut de médecine tropicale (Library of the Institute of Tropical Medicine, Antwerp)
BIUP	Bibliothèque interuniversitaire de pharmacie (Interuniversity Pharmacy Library), Paris
BPITT	Bureau permanent interafricain de la tsé-tsé et de la trypanosomiase (Permanent Inter-African Bureau for Tsetse and Trypanosomiasis)
CAOM	Centre des archives d'outre-mer (Center for Overseas Archives), Aix-en-Provence
CCTA	Commission pour la coopération technique en Afrique (Combined Commission for Technical Co-Operation in Africa South of the Sahara)
FOREAMI	Fonds reine Elizabeth pour l'assistance médicale aux indigènes (Queen Elizabeth Fund for Native Medical Services)
HIV	human immunodeficiency virus
IMTSSA	Institut de médecine tropicale du service de santé des armées (Army Health Service Institute of Tropical Medicine)
IRD	Institut de recherches pour le développement (Development Research Institute)
ISCTR	International Scientific Committee for Trypanosomiasis Research
LSTM	Liverpool School of Tropical Medicine
MB	May & Baker
MRC	Medical Research Council
OCCGE	Organisation de coordination et de coopération pour la lutte contre les grandes endémies (Organization for Coordination and Cooperation in the Control of Major Endemic Diseases)
OCCGEAC	Organisation de coordination et de coopération pour la lutte contre les

	grandes endémies en Afrique centrale (Organization for Coordination and Cooperation in the Control of Major Endemic Diseases in Central Africa)
OCEAC	Organisation de coordination pour la lutte contre les endémies en Afrique centrale (Organization for Coordination of Control of Endemic Diseases in Central Africa)
SAM	Société d'archivage moderne (Society for Modern Archiving)
SFIO	Section française de l'Internationale ouvrière (French Section of the Workers' International)
SGAMS	Service général autonome de la maladie du sommeil (General Autonomous Service for Sleeping Sickness Control)
SGHMP	Service général d'hygiène mobile et de prophylaxie (General Mobile Hygiene and Prophylaxis Services)
SHMP	Service d'hygiène mobile et de prophylaxie (Mobile Hygiene and Prophylaxis Service)
Spécia	Société parisienne d'expansion chimique (Parisian Firm for Chemical Expansion)
UPC	Union des populations du Cameroun (Union of the Peoples of Cameroon)
WHO	World Health Organization

Notes

INTRODUCTION: An Anthropology of Colonial Unreason

1. Translator's note: The expression *mise en valeur*, which has no direct English equivalent, refers to a process of improving the conditions under which resources can be rationally exploited. It prefigured, but was more limited than, what was later referred to as economic development. For a good discussion, see Alice L. Conklin, *A Mission to Civilize: The Republican Idea of Empire in France and West Africa, 1895–1930* (Stanford University Press, Stanford, CA, 1997), 41.

2. Translator's note: This expression refers to the three decades following the end of the Second World War (1946–1975), a period of rapid economic growth and social change in France. See Jean Fourastié, *Les Trente Glorieuses; ou, La révolution invisible de 1946 à 1975* (Fayard, Paris, 1979).

3. Nicolas Hatzfeld and Cédric Lomba, "La grève de Rhodiacéta en 1967," in Dominique Damamme et al. (eds.), *Mai–juin 68* (Éditions de l'Atelier, Paris, 2008), 102–13; Pierre Cayez, *Rhône-Poulenc 1895–1975. Contribution à l'étude d'un groupe industriel* (A. Colin, Masson, Paris, 1988).

4. http://www.archivage-moderne.com.

5. Nancy Rose Hunt, *A Colonial Lexicon: Of Birth Ritual, Medicalization, and Mobility in the Congo* (Duke University Press, Durham, NC, 1999), 24, 324.

6. Ann L. Stoler (ed.), *Imperial Debris: On Ruins and Ruination* (Duke University Press, Durham, NC, 2013). On the relationship between modernization and decolonization in France during the Trente Glorieuses, see, for example, Kristin Ross, *Fast Cars, Clean Bodies: Decolonization and the Reordering of French Culture* (MIT Press, Cambridge, MA, 1995).

7. Lomidine is the French brand name of the drug, which was also trademarked under the name of Pentamidine, notably in the United Kingdom. The generic name pentamidine (uncapitalized) designates the active compound (4,4–diamidino-alpha,omega-diphenoxypentane), which can be formulated as various salts (such as pentamidine diisethionate or dimesilate); the formula has varied since the 1930s. In this book, I alternate between Pentamidine and Lomidine to designate the commercial drug according to national context, and I use pentamidine when I am referring to the compound itself.

8. René Labusquière, *Santé rurale et médecine préventive en Afrique. Stratégie à opposer aux principales affections* (Imprimerie Saint-Paul, Bar-le-Duc, France, 1974), 260.

9. Gaston Bachelard, *L'engagement rationaliste* (Presses Universitaires de France, Paris, 1972), 141. On retrospective judgment as a narrative and heuristic device in the history of science, see Dominique Pestre, *Introduction aux sciences studies* (La Découverte, Paris, 2006), 42.

10. Notably, pentamidine can cause a malignant ventricular arrhythmia called "torsades de pointes," which can lead to cardiac arrest. See A. Gonzalez et al., "Pentamidine-Induced Torsade de Pointes," *American Heart Journal* 122.5 (1991), 1489–92.

11. Frederick Cooper, *Colonialism in Question: Theory, Knowledge, History* (University of California Press, Berkeley, 2005), 17.

12. For a social scientific approach to the agency of things, see, for example, Bruno Latour, *Reassembling the Social: An Introduction to Actor-Network-Theory* (Oxford University Press, Oxford, 2005), 70–82.

13. *Trypanosoma brucei* has several subspecies. The form prevalent in West and Central Africa is *T. gambiense*, while *T. rhodesiense* is prevalent in East Africa.

14. Catherine Coquery-Vidrovitch, "Evolution démographique de l'Afrique coloniale," in Marc Ferro (ed.), *Le livre noir du colonialisme, XVI–XXIe siècle. De l'extermination à la repentance* (Robert Laffont, Paris, 2003), 557–66; Jean-Pierre Chrétien, "La crise écologique de l'Afrique orientale au début du XXe siècle. Le cas de l'Imbo au Burundi entre 1890 et 1916," in *Questions sur la paysannerie au Burundi* (Université du Burundi/Centre de Recherches Africaines [Paris I], Paris, 1987).

15. Michael Worboys, "The Emergence of Tropical Medicine: A Study in the Establishment of a Scientific Speciality," in Gérard Lemaine et al. (eds.), *Perspectives on the Emergence of Scientific Disciplines* (Mouton, Paris, 1976), 75–98; Maryinez Lyons, *The Colonial Disease: A Social History of Sleeping Sickness in Northern Zaire, 1900–1940* (Cambridge University Press, Cambridge, 1992); Deborah Joy Neill, *Networks in Tropical Medicine: Internationalism, Colonialism, and the Rise of a Medical Specialty, 1890–1930* (Stanford University Press, Stanford, CA, 2012).

16. This is illustrated, for example, by the reception of a movie on the Jamot Mission presented at the Paris Colonial Exhibition. See Béatrice de Pastre, "Cinéma éducateur et propagande coloniale à Paris au début des années 1930," *Revue d'Histoire Moderne et Contemporaine* 51.4 (2004), 135–51.

17. Michael Worboys, "The Comparative History of Sleeping Sickness in East and Central Africa, 1900–1914," *History of Science* 32 (1994), 89–102; Ann Beck, "Medicine and Society in Tanganyika, 1890–1930: A Historical Inquiry," *Transactions of the American Philosophical Society* 67.3 (1977), 1–59; Jean-Paul Bado, *Les grandes endémies en Afrique, 1900–1960* (Karthala, Paris, 1996); Jean-Paul Bado, *Eugène Jamot, 1879–1937. Le médecin de la maladie du sommeil ou trypanosomiase* (Karthala, Paris, 2011); Lyons, *The Colonial Disease*; Rita Headrick, *Colonialism, Health and Illness in French Equatorial Africa, 1885–1935* (African Studies Association Press, Atlanta, GA, 1994); Jean-Pierre Dozon, "Quand les pastoriens traquaient la maladie du sommeil," *Sciences Sociales et Santé* 3.3–4 (1985), 27–56; Danielle Domergue-Cloarec, *La santé en Côte d'Ivoire, 1905–1958*, 2 vols. (Publications de l'Université de Toulouse le Mirail, Toulouse, 1986); Helen Tilley, *Africa as a Living Laboratory: Empire, Development, and the Problem of Scientific Knowledge, 1870–1950* (University of Chicago Press, Chicago, 2011).

18. Guillaume Lachenal, "Le médecin qui voulut être roi. Médecine coloniale et utopie au Cameroun," *Annales Histoire, Sciences Sociales* 65.1 (2010), 121–56; Kirk Arden Hoppe, *Lords of the Fly: Sleeping Sickness Control in British East Africa, 1900–1960* (Praeger, London, 2003).

19. L. Lapeyssonnie, *La médecine coloniale. Mythe et réalités* (Seghers, Paris, 1984). For a study of African auxiliaries in the health service in Cameroon, see Wang Sonne, "Les auxilliaires autochtones dans l'action sanitaire publique au Cameroun sous administration française (1916–1945)," doctoral thesis, Université de Yaoundé, 1983.

20. Jean Suret-Canale, *Afrique noire occidentale et centrale*, vol. 2: *L'ère coloniale, 1900–1945* (Éditions Sociales, Paris, 1958), 510.

21. Michel Foucault, *Histoire de la sexualité*, vol. 1: *La volonté de savoir* (Gallimard, Paris, 1976), 183. On the links between German tropical medicine and the Nazi politics of racial hygiene, see Wolfgang U. Eckart, *Medizin und Kolonialimperialismus. Deutschland 1884–1945* (F. Schöningh, Paderborn, 1997); Guillaume Lachenal, "Médecine, comparaisons et échanges inter-impériaux dans le mandat Camerounais. Une histoire croisée franco-allemande de la Mission Jamot," *Bulletin Canadien d'Histoire de la Médecine* 30.2 (2013), 23–45.

22. http://www.ted.com/talks/niall_ferguson_the_6_killer_apps_of_prosperity,   accessed April 22, 2016.

23. Guillaume Lachenal and Bertrand Taithe, "Une généalogie missionaire et coloniale de l'humanitaire. Le cas Aujoulat au Cameroun, 1935–1973," *Mouvement Social* 227 (2009), 45–63.

24. Two twenty-first-century biomedical studies are well researched: Jacques Pepin, *The Origins of AIDS* (Cambridge University Press, Cambridge, 2011), 156–57; and G. Ollivier and D. Legros, "Trypanosomiase humaine africaine. Historique de la thérapeutique et de ses échecs," *Tropical Medicine and International Health* 6.11 (2001), 855–63.

25. For historiographical reviews of the field, see Warwick Anderson, "How's the Empire? An Essay Review," *Journal of the History of Medicine and Allied Sciences* 58 (2003), 459–65; Karine Delaunay, "Faire de la santé un lieu pour l'histoire de l'Afrique. Essai d'historiographie," *Outre-Mers* 93.346–47 (2005), 7–46; Nancy Rose Hunt, "Health and Healing," in John Parker and Richard J. Reid (eds.), *The Oxford Handbook of Modern African History* (Oxford University Press, Oxford, 2013), 378–95.

26. Michel Foucault mentions briefly the "feedback effects" of colonialism in the European world in Foucault, *"Il faut défendre la société." Cours au Collége de France (1975–1976)* (Seuil/Gallimard, Paris, 1997), 89. The approach to colonies as "laboratories of modernity" was developed by Paul Rabinow, *Une France si moderne. Naissance du social, 1800–1950* (Buchet-Chastel, Paris, 2005), 289–317; and taken up by a considerable body of recent work. For an overview, see Lachenal, "Le médecin qui voulut être roi."

27. Frederick Cooper, *Decolonization and African Society: The Labor Question in French and British Africa* (Cambridge University Press, Cambridge, 1996).

28. Achille Mbembe, *La naissance du maquis dans le Sud Cameroun, 1920–1960* (Karthala, Paris, 1996), 33.

29. Bruno Latour, *Pasteur. Guerre et paix des microbes. Suivi de irréductions* (La Découverte, Paris, 2001).

30. For examples of Africans' interpretations of colonial medicine, see Luise White, *Speaking with Vampires: Rumor and History in Colonial Africa* (University of California Press, Berkeley, 2000); Hunt, *A Colonial Lexicon*.

31. On medical bêtise in the work of Flaubert, see, for example, Norioki Sugaya, *Flaubert épistémologue. Autour du dossier médical de "Bouvard et Pécuchet"* (Rodopi, Amsterdam, 2010). The issue of medical bêtise in the colonial context arises regularly in the work of Louis-Ferdinand Céline: Céline, *Voyage au bout de la nuit* (Denoël et Steele, Paris, 1932); Céline, *L'église* (Denoël et Steele, Paris, 1933).

32. Even some highly respected studies can be accused of this, for example, Elsa Dorlin, *La matrice de la race. Généalogie coloniale et sexuelle de la nation française* (La Découverte, Paris, 2006).

33. Achille Mbembe, "Faut-il provincialiser la France?" *Politique Africaine* 119 (2010), 159–88, 182.

34. Ibid.

35. Londa L. Schiebinger, *Plants and Empire: Colonial Bioprospecting in the Atlantic World* (Harvard University Press, Cambridge, MA, 2004); Ann L. Stoler, *Along the Archival Grain: Epistemic Anxieties and Colonial Common Sense* (Princeton University Press, Princeton, NJ, 2008).

36. Johannes Fabian, *Out of Our Minds: Reason and Madness in the Exploration of Central Africa* (University of California Press, Berkeley, 2000), 281.

37. Warwick Anderson, *Colonial Pathologies: American Tropical Medicine, Race and Hygiene in the Philippines* (Duke University Press, Durham, NC, 2006), 9, 74–103; Nancy Rose Hunt, *A Nervous State: Violence, Remedies, and Reverie in Colonial Congo* (Duke University Press, Durham, NC, 2016).

38. Eric Jennings, *Curing the Colonizers: Hydrotherapy, Climatology, and French Colonial Spas* (Duke University Press, Durham, NC, 2006).

39. Fabian, *Out of Our Minds*.

40. Stoler, *Along the Archival Grain*, 254.

41. Jean-Baptiste Fressoz, *L'apocalypse joyeuse. Une histoire du risque technologique* (Seuil, Paris, 2012), 15

42. Cooper, *Decolonization and African Society*, 451.

43. See, for example, Jacques Derrida, *The Beast and the Sovereign* (Chicago: University of Chicago Press, 2010), 222–23. See also Magdalena Cámpora, "La *bêtise*, un privilège français?" *Flaubert* 6 (2011), http://flaubert.revues.org/1651, accessed January 15, 2016.

44. Isabelle Stengers, *In Catastrophic Times: Resisting the Coming Barbarism*, trans. Andrew Goffey (London, Open Humanities Press and Meson Press), 115.

45. Alain Roger, *Bréviaire de la bêtise* (Gallimard, Paris, 2008), 30–31.

46. George Orwell, *Burmese Days* (1934; rpt., Penguin, London, 2009), 121.

47. For an overview of the philosophical problem of bêtise, notably in the work of Nietzsche and Deleuze, see Roger, *Bréviaire de la bêtise*. On the Flaubertian issue of bêtise and how it is discussed by Barthes, see Anne Herschberg-Pierrot (ed.), *Flaubert, l'empire de la bêtise* (Nouvelles Cecile Défaut, Nantes, 2011).

48. Jean-Marc Lévy-Leblond, "Le miroir, la cornue et la pierre de touche; ou, Que peut la littérature pour la science?" *Cahiers de Narratologie* 18 (June 28, 2010), https://narratologie.revues.org/6002, accessed January 3, 2017.

49. Richard C. Keller, *Colonial Madness: Psychiatry in French North Africa* (University of Chicago Press, Chicago, 2007); Fabian, *Out of Our Minds*; Bertrand Taithe, *The Killer Trail: A Colonial Scandal in the Heart of Africa* (Oxford University Press, Oxford, 2009).

50. Didier Fassin, "Le culturalisme pratique de la santé publique. Critique d'un sens commun," in Jean Pierre Dozon and Didier Fassin (eds.), *Critique de la santé publique. Une approche anthropologique* (Balland, Paris, 2001), 181–208; Paul Farmer, *Infections and Inequalities: The Modern Plagues* (University of California Press, Berkeley, 1999), 228–61.

51. On "stupid deaths," see Paul Farmer, *Pathologies of Power: Health, Human Rights, and the New War on the Poor* (University of California Press, Berkeley, 2003), 144.

52. Stengers, *In Catastrophic Times*, 120, 122.

53. Paul Veyne, *Writing History: Essay on Epistemology* (Manchester University Press, Manchester, England, 1984), 184.

54. Roland Barthes, "La division des langages" (1973), in his *Oeuvres complètes*, vol. 4 (Le Seuil, Paris, 2002), 348–60, 350, cited in Anne Herschberg-Pierrot, "Roland Barthes, la bêtise et Flaubert," in Herschberg-Pierrot, *Flaubert, l'empire de la bêtise*, 333–56, 339–41.

55. Roland Barthes, *S/Z* (1970), in his *Oeuvres complètes*, vol. 3 (Le Seuil, Paris, 2002), 119–346, 291.

56. Jean Dutertre, "Jean-Marc et la trypano," http://perso.orange.fr/jdtr, accessed September 2, 2013.

57. Teju Cole, "The White-Savior Industrial Complex," March 21, 2012, http://www.theatlantic.com/international/archive/2012/03/the-white-savior-industrial-complex/254843, accessed May 30, 2016.

58. Susan Sontag, "At the Same Time: The Novelist and Moral Reasoning," in her *At the Same Time: Essays and Speeches* (Hamish Hamilton, London, 2007), 210–31, 225–28.

59. For example, see Robert Bud, *Penicillin: Triumph and Tragedy* (Oxford University Press, Oxford, 2007); John E. Lesch, *The First Miracle Drugs: How the Sulfa Drugs Transformed Medicine* (Oxford University Press, Oxford, 2007). My approach is biographical in the sense that I address a drug as a character, with its own name (trademark) and biomedical identity (active ingredients). The

biographical approach to pharmaceuticals has been deployed somewhat differently by anthropologists who, following Arjun Appadurai, use it to trace the "life cycle" of medicines as commodities, from their production to their consumption. See Susan Reynolds Whyte, Sjaak van der Geest, and Anita Hardon, *Social Lives of Medicines* (Cambridge University Press, Cambridge, 2002); Sjaak van der Geest, Susan Reynolds Whyte, and Anita Hardon, "The Anthropology of Pharmaceuticals: A Biographical Approach," *Annual Review of Anthropology* 25 (1996), 153–78.

CHAPTER 1: The Wonder Drug

1. Bruno Strasser, "Magic Bullets and Wonder Pills: Making Drugs and Diseases in the Twentieth Century," *Historical Studies in the Natural Sciences* 38.2 (2008), 302–12. For tales of the discovery of pentamidine, see David Greenwood, *Antimicrobial Drugs: Chronicle of a Twentieth Century Medical Triumph* (Oxford University Press, Oxford, 2008), 282–83; Fred Lembeck, "Successful Errors and Other Odd Ways to New Discoveries," *Medical History* 11.2 (1967), 157–64, 163; Walter Sneader, *Drug Discovery: A History* (Wiley, Hoboken, NJ, 2005), 277.

2. I am grateful to Dora Vargha for this information.

3. N. von Jancso and H. von Jancso, "Chemotherapische Wirkung und Kohlehydratstoffwechsel: die Heilwirkung von Guanidinderivativaten auf die Trypanosomeinfektion," *Zeitschrift für Immunitätforsch* 86 (1935).

4. Helen J. Power, *Tropical Medicine in the Twentieth Century: A History of the Liverpool School of Tropical Medicine, 1898–1990* (Kegan Paul International, London, 1999).

5. E. M. Lourie and W. Yorke, "Studies in Chemotherapy. XVI: The Trypanocidal Action of Synthalin," *Annals of Tropical Medicine and Parasitology* 31.3 (1937), 435–45.

6. H. King, E. M. Lourie, and W. Yorke, "New Trypanocidal Substances," *Lancet* 233 (1937), 1360.

7. Greenwood, *Antimicrobial Drugs*, 282–83.

8. The term "therapeutic revolution" is in debate among historians; see John E. Lesch, *The First Miracle Drugs: How the Sulfa Drugs Transformed Medicine* (Oxford University Press, Oxford, 2007), 4.

9. Jean-Paul Gaudillière, "Introduction: Drug Trajectories," *Studies in History and Philosophy of Biological and Biomedical Sciences* 36.4 (2005), 603–611; Jean-Paul Gaudillière, *Inventer la biomédecine. La France, l'Amérique et la production des savoirs du vivant (1945–1965)* (La Découverte, Paris, 2002).

10. In the early twentieth century, "chemotherapy" referred to a field of research dedicated to the study of synthetic therapeutic compounds. It did not yet have the more restricted meaning of cancer treatment that it now has in popular usage.

11. Deborah Neill, "Paul Ehrlich's Colonial Connections: Scientific Networks and the Response to the Sleeping Sickness Epidemic, 1900–1914," *Social History of Medicine* 22.1 (2009), 61–77.

12. Établissements Poulenc frères, *La maladie du sommeil* (Éditions EPF, Paris, 1927).

13. On colonial Indochina, see Laurence Monnais, "From Colonial Medicines to Global Pharmaceuticals? The Introduction of Sulfa Drugs in French Vietnam," *East Asian Science: Technology and Society* 3 (2009), 257–85; on Africa, see Luise White, *Speaking with Vampires: Rumor and History in Colonial Africa* (University of California Press, Berkeley, 2000), 100–101.

14. Jennifer Beinart, "The Inner World of Imperial Sickness: The MRC and Research in Tropical Medicine," in Joan Austoker and Linda Bryder (eds.), *Historical Perspectives on the Role of the MRC Essays in the History of the Medical Research Council of the United Kingdom and Its Predecessor, the Medical Research Committee, 1913–1953* (Oxford University Press, Oxford, 1989).

15. Viviane Quirke, *Collaboration in the Pharmaceutical Industry: Changing Relationships in Britain and France, 1935–1965* (Routledge, New York, 2008), 36–40.

16. Ibid., 81.

17. Henry Dale, cited in Warrington Yorke, "Recent Work on the Chemotherapy of Protozoal Infections," *Transactions of the Royal Society of Tropical Medicine and Hygiene* 33.5 (1940), 463–82, 479.

18. These are so-called aromatic diamidines, because they contain two rings derived from benzene, each containing an amidine group, linked together by a carbon chain of variable nature and length (five in the case of pentamidine).

19. LSTM, TM/13 June–4 January, "Correspondence Relating to Research Funding from May & Baker Limited: Chemotherapy Arrangements" (June 1938).

20. A dozen articles were published between 1937 and 1940, most authored by Emanuel Lourie.

21. LSTM, TM/13 June–4 January, Arthur Ewins, letter to Emanuel Lourie, October 4, 1945.

22. Power, *Tropical Medicine in the Twentieth Century*, 79–103.

23. Charles Morley Wenyon, "Warrington Yorke, 1883–1943," *Obituary Notices of Fellows of the Royal Society* 4.13 (1944), 523–45.

24. F. Glyn-Hugues, Emanuel Lourie, and Warrington Yorke, "Studies in Chemotherapy. XVII: The Action of Undecan Diamidine in Malaria," *Annals of Tropical Medicine and Parasitology* 32.1 (1938), 103–7.

25. Warrington Yorke, "The Therapeutic Action of the Aromatic Diamidines in the Treatment of Protozoal Infections of Man and Stock," *British Medical Bulletin* 2.3–4 (1944), 60–64, 61.

26. LSTM, "The Incorporated Liverpool School of Tropical Medicine, Fortieth Annual Report, August 1, 1938–July 31, 1939," 1939, 3.

27. Power, *Tropical Medicine in the Twentieth Century*, 51–72.

28. LSTM, TM18/3/75, Warrington Yorke, letter to Thomas Davey, May 23, 1939.

29. Born in South Africa, Emanuel Lourie (1904–56) studied medicine at University College Hospital in London and worked in Chicago and in Palestine before joining the Liverpool School of Tropical Medicine. F. Hawking, "Dr. E. M. Lourie," *Nature* 178.4533 (1956), 569–70; LSTM, TM18/3/75, Davey, letter to Yorke, April 23, 1939.

30. LSTM, TM18/3/75, Thomas Davey, letters to Yorke, May 25 and 30, 1939.

31. LSTM, TM/18/3/35, Colonel Gaston Muraz, letter to Professor Davey, September 25, 1939.

32. LSTM, TM/18/3/35, Thomas Davey and Emanuel Lourie, "Report on a Sleeping Sickness Survey of the Eastern Border of Sierra Leone," 1939.

33. LSTM, TM18/3/75, Davey, letter to Yorke, August 8, 1939.

34. Davey and Lourie, "Report on a Sleeping Sickness Survey," 6.

35. E. M. Lourie, "Treatment of Sleeping Sickness in Sierra Leone," *Annals of Tropical Medicine and Parasitology* 36 (1942), 113–31.

36. LSTM, TM/14/4/12, *Daily Mail*, August 14, 1939; *Manchester Dispatch*, August 14, 1939, Newspaper Cuttings, 1938–1941.

37. LSTM, TM18/3/75, Warrington Yorke, letter to Davey, December 13, 1939.

38. See the correspondence collected in LSTM, TM18/3/75.

39. LSTM, TM18/3/75, Thomas Davey, letter to Yorke, November 21, 1939.

40. For example, see J.-L. McLetchie, "The Treatment of Early Cases of Nigerian Trypanosomiasis with 4:4'diamidino stilbene," *Annals of Tropical Medicine and Parasitology* 34 (1940), 73–82.

41. Yorke, "Recent Work on the Chemotherapy of Protozoal Infections."

42. Ibid., 473.

43. Ibid., 474.

44. T. L. Lawson, "Trypanosomiasis Treated with 'Pentamidine,'" *Lancet* 2 (1942), 480–83. Scratching is discussed by G. F. T. Saunders, "Preliminary Report on the Treatment of Sleeping Sickness by 4:4'diamidino diphenoxpentane," *Annals of Tropical Medicine and Parasitology* 35 (1941), 169–86.

45. G. McComas and N. H. Martin, "Trypanosomiasis Treated with Pentamidine: A Fatal Case," *Lancet* 1 (1944), 338–39.

46. Lourie, "Treatment of Sleeping Sickness."

47. C. Bowesman, "A Short Report of the Use of 4:4'-diaminidino stilben in the Treatment of Human Sleeping Sickness," *Annals of Tropical Medicine and Parasitology* 34 (1940), 217–22; R. D. Harding, "A Trial with 4:4'-diamidino stilbene in the Treatment of Sleeping Sickness at Gadau, Northern Nigeria," *Annals of Tropical Medicine and Parasitology* 34 (1940), 101–5; R. D. Harding, "The Influence of Sleeping Sickness on Mortality in Two Districts of Northern Nigeria," *Transactions of the Royal Society of Tropical Medicine and Hygiene* 33.5 (1940), 483–500; McLetchie, "Treatment of Early Cases"; Saunders, "Preliminary Report on the Treatment of Sleeping Sickness."

48. R. R. Bomford, "Trypanosomiasis in a European Treated with Pentamidine," *British Medical Journal* 2 (1944), 276–77.

49. Wenyon, "Warrington Yorke."

50. Henry Dale, "A Prospect in Therapeutics," *British Medical Journal* 2 (1943), 411–16.

CHAPTER 2: Experiments without Borders

1. Warwick Anderson, "Where Is the Postcolonial History of Medicine?" *Bulletin of the History of Medicine* 72.3 (1998), 522–30.

2. Translator's note: Many staff members of the colonial French and Belgian medical services were military personnel. They were referred to by composite military-medical titles (for example, Colonel-Doctor, Lieutenant-Pharmacist). Since there is no equivalent in English, these titles have been translated literally.

3. AA, 4464/923, L. Van Hoof, letter to Dr. Ewins, June 30, 1943.

4. J. Rhodain, "Nécrologie. Lucien Van Hoof," *Annales de Société Belge de Médecine Tropicale* 28 (1948), 381–84; A. C. Thomas, "Hommage au Docteur L. Van Hoof," *Annales de Société Belge de Médecine Tropicale* 34.5 (1954), 559–63; Académie Royale des Sciences d'Outre-Mer and M. Kivits, "Van Hoof," *Biographie Belge d'Outre-Mer* 6 (1968), 503–6.

5. Louis Pierquin, *Historique du laboratoire médicale et de Institut de médecine tropicale Princesse Astrid à Léopoldville* (Graphicongo, Léopoldville, 1958); Myriam Mertens, "Chemical Compounds in the Congo: Pharmaceuticals and the 'Crossed History' of Public Health in Belgian Africa (ca. 1905–1939)," PhD diss., University of Ghent, 2014.

6. L. Van Hoof, C. Henrard, and E. Peel, "Pentamidine in the Prevention and Treatment of Trypanosomiasis," *Transactions of the Royal Society of Tropical Medicine and Hygiene* 37.4 (1944), 271–80.

7. AA, 4464/923, L. Van Hoof, letter to Dr. Forgan, June 30, 1943.

8. Nancy Rose Hunt, *A Colonial Lexicon: Of Birth Ritual, Medicalization, and Mobility in the Congo* (Duke University Press, Durham, NC, 1999), 95–96, 209.

9. J.-D. Fulton, "The Prophylactic Action of Various Aromatic Diamidines in Trypanosomiases of Mice," *Annals of Tropical Medicine and Parasitology* 38.1 (1944), 78–84.

10. In the 1930s, several methods were developed in England and in Africa to improve the control of experimental trypanosome infection; some sought to quantify the "infective power" of tsetse flies in the lab, while others resorted to injections of infected blood from monkey, guinea pigs, and humans. H. L. Duke, "On the Prophylactic Action of 'Bayer 205' against the Trypanosoma of Man," *Lancet* 1 (1936), 463–69.

11. L. Van Hoof, C. Henrard, and E. Peel, "Chimioprophylaxie de la maladie du sommeil par la pentamidine," *Annales de Société Belge de Médecine Tropicale* 26 (1946), 371–84.

12. "The controls," specified Dr. Lewillon, the Belgian doctor responsible for this trial, "were chosen in a way to spread the risks of infection as evenly as possible in both of the experimental groups (a woman or child control in each large family)." Retrospectively, it can be noted that this protocol introduced an age difference between the groups (there were about twice as many children in the control group). The data from 1942 show that nearly 40 percent of the new infections before the experiment were in children. This simple fact of overrepresenting children is enough to explain the final results of the trial (unfortunately, we do not have information on the ages of the control subjects who were found to be infected). AA, RA/MED45, Dr. Lewillon, "Rapport annuel 1942," 22.

13. Ibid., 29.

14. L. Van Hoof et al., "A Field Experiment on the Prophylactic Value of Pentamidine in Sleeping Sicknesss," *Transactions of the Royal Society of Tropical Medicine and Hygiene* 39.4 (1946), 327–29, 329.

15. F. Van Den Branden, "Sur un essai d'administration de Bayer 205 prophylactique dans une agglomération indigène," *Annales de Société Belge de Médecine Tropicale* 5 (1925), 175–77.

16. H. de Marqueissac, "Contribution à l'emploi du Moranyl (205 Bayer, 309 Fourneau) donné à titre préventif dans la trypanosomiase humaine (secteur de Pagouda, Togo)," *Bulletin de la Société de Pathologie Exotique* 25 (1932), 347–53; C. Wilcocks, J.-F. Corson, and R. L. Sheppard, *A Survey of Recent Work on Trypanosomiasis and Tsetse Flies*, vol. 1 (Bureau of Hygiene and Tropical Diseases, London, 1946), 69; Eugène Jamot and Marcel Chambon, "Contribution à l'étude du pouvoir préventif du 205 Bayer–309 Fourneau, contre la maladie du sommeil," *Bulletin de la Société de Pathologie Exotique* 23 (1930), 491–99.

17. Lewillon, "Rapport annuel 1942," 22.

18. Van Hoof, Henrard, and Peel, "Chimioprophylaxie," 381.

19. Lewillon, "Rapport annuel 1942," 29.

20. Van Hoof, Henrard, and Peel, "Chimioprophylaxie," 381.

21. Direction du service de l'hygiène—Léopoldville—Congo belge, "Recueil de travaux de sciences médicales au Congo belge," 1942, 1.

22. AA, 4464/923, Congo belge, Service de l'information, "La pénicilline au Congo belge," 1944.

23. AA, 4464/923, telegram, January 13, 1944.

24. Service de l'information, "La pénicilline au Congo belge."

25. L. Van Hoof, "Observations on Trypanosomiasis in the Belgian Congo," *Transactions of the Royal Society of Tropical Medicine and Hygiene* 40.6 (1947), 728–54, 741.

26. C. C. Chesterman et al., "[Ordinary Meeting, 20th February 1947, Discussion]," *Transactions of the Royal Society of Tropical Medicine and Hygiene* 40.6 (1947), 755–61, 755.

27. LSTM, excerpt from Dr. Thomas Davey's travel diary.

28. Colonel Gaston Muraz, "Des très larges mesures de chimioprophylaxie par injections intramusculaires de diamidines aromatiques (lomidine) mises en œuvre depuis plusieurs années déjà et tendant à l'éradication de la maladie du sommeil dans les territoires de l'Afrique noire française (AOF, AEF, Cameroun et Togo sous mandat), contaminés de cette endémie," *Bulletin de l'Académie Nationale de Médecine* 138.33–35 (1954), 614–17, 615. Translator's note: Given the length and informative content of this title, here is a translation: "Chemoprophylaxis Measures by Intramuscular Injections of Aromatic Diamidines (Lomidine), Which Have Already Been Implemented on a Vast Scale in the Last Few Years, Are Leading towards the Eradication of Sleeping Sickness in the Territories of French Black Africa (AOF, AEF, Cameroon, and Togo under Mandate), Contaminated by This Epidemic."

29. J. Le Rouzic and L. Lapeyssonnie, "Les médicaments nouveaux dans la trypanosomiase," *Bulletin Médical de l'AOF* 5.1 (1948), 7–22, 18.

30. L. Nodenot, "Le traitement de la trypanosomiase par les médicaments nouveaux," *Bulletin Médical de l'AOF* 4.1 (1947), 73–74.

31. LSTM, TM/14/5/Davey/6, Thomas Davey, travel diary, July 15, 1945.

32. Louis-Ferdinand Céline, *L'église* (Denoël et Steele, Paris, 1933). Translator's note: Louis-Ferdinand Céline was the pen name of the author and physician Louis Ferdinand Auguste Destouches. Several of his novels satirized colonial society as well as the medical profession.

33. G. Saleun and J. Chassain, "Essai de chimioprophylaxie de la trypanosomiase humaine en Afrique équatoriale française par la pentamidine," *Bulletin de la Société de Pathologie Exotique* 41 (1948), 165.

34. Viviane Quirke, "Experiments in Collaboration: The Changing Relationship between Scientists and Pharmaceutical Companies in Britain and in France, 1935–1965," DPhil. thesis, University of Oxford, 1999, 44–46; Pierre Cayez, *Rhône-Poulenc 1895–1975. Contribution à l'étude d'un groupe industriel* (A. Colin, Masson, Paris, 1988); Judy Slinn, *A History of May & Baker: 1834–1984* (Hobsons, Cambridge, 1984).

35. Cayez, *Rhône-Poulenc*, 126–27.

36. Léon Launoy and Henri Lagodsky, "De l'action préventive contre les trypanosomoses expérimentales de certaines diamidines aromatiques, en particulier du diamidino-diphénoxypentane," *Journal de Physiologie* 39.1 (1946), 49–58.

37. Quirke, "Experiments in Collaboration," 145n57.

38. Arch. Spécia, box 831362B123, Direction recherche thérapeutique, letter to Spécia Saint-Fons, December 7, 1944; Direction scientifique Spécia, letter to DG Spécia and Saint-Fons, December 11, 1945.

39. Marcel Guillot, "Léon Launoy (1876–1971)," *Bulletin de l'Académie Nationale de Médecine* 156.14 (1972), 452–62.

40. Jacques Pierre Ziegler, "Contribution à l'étude de la chimioprophylaxie de la maladie du sommeil, no. 313," thesis for doctorate in medicine, Faculté de médecine de Paris, 1948, 97.

41. Léon Launoy and Henri Lagodsky, "Documents relatifs à l'activité trypanocide de quelques diamidines," *Bulletin de la Société de Pathologie Exotique* 33 (1940), 320–24.

42. Léon Launoy and Henri Lagodsky, "De l'action préventive d'une diamidine aromatique, la diamidino-diphénoxypentane, sur deux trypanosomoses expérimentales du rat," *Bulletin de la Société de Pathologie Exotique* 39 (1946), 160–67, 161.

43. Caroline Chareton, "Le legs Launoy. Trypanosomoses africaines. De Jamot, homme de terrain, à Launoy, homme de laboratoire," professional practice thesis in pharmacy, Université de Caen, 2004, 18; R. Arnaud, "Au sujet du Moranyl. Deux opérations de moralynisation dans le Moyen-Congo," *Bulletin de la Société de Pathologie Exotique* 22 (1929), 872–80.

44. Léon Launoy, "Sur l'importance du problème des trypanosomiases en Afrique équatoriale," *Annales Coloniales Quotidiennes* (October 17, 1929), reprinted in Léon Launoy, *Recherches sur les trypanosomoses expérimentales, index bibliographique, hypothèses de travail, 1926–1949* (M. Declume, Lons-le-Saunier, 1949), 121.

45. Léon Launoy, "La prophylaxie chimique dans la lutte contre la maladie du sommeil," *Annales Coloniales Quotidiennes* (December 1929), reprinted in Launoy, *Recherches sur les trypanosomoses expérimentales*, 126.

46. Léon Launoy, "Instruire l'autochtone," *Annales Coloniales Quotidiennes* (August 4, 1928), reprinted in Launoy, *Recherches sur les trypanosomoses expérimentales*.

47. Douglas M. Haynes, *Imperial Medicine: Patrick Manson and the Conquest of Tropical Disease* (University of Pennsylvania Press, Philadelphia, 2001).

48. Léon Launoy, *Éléments de physiologie humaine* (Maloine, Paris, 1947).

49. Léon Launoy, "Aperçu sur les origines, les caractères, le but et l'avenir de la thérapeutique chimique étiologique," *Biologie Médicale* 37.9–10 (1948).

50. Launoy, "La prophylaxie chimique," reprinted in Launoy, *Recherches sur les trypanosomoses expérimentales*, 123.

51. Léon Launoy, "Sur quelques difficultés de l'application clinique des résultats expérimentaux relatifs au traitement des trypanosomoses, et sur la thérapie synergique de ces infections. Leçon au Collège de France," *Biologie Médicale* 26.4 (1936), reprinted in Launoy, *Recherches sur les trypanosomoses expérimentales*.

52. Ibid.

53. Ibid. Launoy's original definition of chemoprophylaxis was given in 1929 and reiterated in numerous articles on pentamidine.

54. Léon Launoy, "À propos de la prophylaxie chimique de quelques trypanosomoses expérimentales," *Bulletin de l'Académie Nationale de Médecine* 133.31–32 (1949), 617–20, 620. Mathis's comments are found in the discussion following the article.

55. Launoy, *Recherches sur les trypanosomoses expérimentales*.

56. Arch. Spécia, box 831362B123, December 4, 1946.

57. Stovarsol, an arsenical drug used to treat syphilis, was named for its inventor, Ernest Fourneau, on the basis of the English translation of his last name, which means "stove" in French (the same approach was used for stovacaine, a local anesthetic). Daniel Bovet, *Une chimie qui guérit. Histoire de la découverte des sulfamides* (Payot, Paris, 1988).

58. Arch. Spécia, box 831362B123, Direction technique, January 29, 1947.

59. Muraz, "Des très larges mesures," 616.

CHAPTER 3: The New Deal of Colonial Medicine

1. W. Eraerts, "La propamidine comme préventif dans deux foyers de trypanosomiase humaine au Congo belge," *Annales de Société Belge de Médecine Tropicale* 27 (1947), 201, 212.

2. L. Van Hoof, "Observations on Trypanosomiasis in the Belgian Congo," *Transactions of the Royal Society of Tropical Medicine and Hygiene* 40.6 (1947), 740.

3. Bruno Latour, *Pasteur. Guerre et paix des microbes. Suivi de irréductions* (La Découverte, Paris, 2001). See also, on the coproduction of "context" in history, Latour, *Changer de société, refaire de la sociologie* (La Découverte, Paris, 2006), 107–8.

4. Frederick Cooper, *Africa since 1940: The Past of the Present* (Cambridge University Press, Cambridge, 2003); Christophe Bonneuil, "Development as Experiment," *Osiris* 14 (2001), 258–81; Helen Tilley, *Africa as a Living Laboratory: Empire, Development, and the Problem of Scientific Knowledge, 1870–1950* (University of Chicago Press, Chicago, 2011).

5. Foucault used the term "biopolitics" (*biopolitique*) to define the political management of a population as a biological entity. For Foucault, biopolitics is one of two dimensions of the "power over life" (biopower) wielded by modern states beginning in the eighteenth century. The other is "anatomo-politics," referring to the disciplining of individual bodies. Michel Foucault, *"Il faut défendre la société." Cours au Collège de France (1975–1976)* (Seuil/Gallimard, Paris, 1997), 213–34; Michel Foucault, *Histoire de la sexualité*, vol. 1: *La volonté de savoir* (Gallimard, Paris, 1976), 177–91.

6. Vincent Bonnecase, *La pauvreté au Sahel. Du savoir colonial à la mesure internationale* (Karthala, Paris, 2011); Frederick Cooper, *Decolonization and African Society: The Labor Question in French and British Africa* (Cambridge University Press, Cambridge, 1996).

7. Sunil S. Amrith, *Decolonizing International Health: India and Southeast Asia, 1930–1965* (Palgrave Macmillan, Basingstoke, England, 2006).

8. IMTSSA, box 111, Médecin-colonel Farinaud, "Rapport annuel. Année 1944" (1945), 242.

9. Jean-Pierre Dozon, "Quand les pastoriens traquaient la maladie du sommeil," *Sciences Sociales et Santé* 3.3–4 (1985), 27–56.

10. Randall M. Packard, "Malaria Dreams: Postwar Visions of Health and Development in the Third World," *Medical Anthropology* 17.3 (1997), 279–96.

11. "La santé publique dans le 2e plan d'équipement et de modernisation des territoires d'outre-mer," *Médecine Tropicale* 14.3 (1954), 204–32, 211.

12. Nancy Stepan, *Eradication: Ridding the World of Diseases Forever?* (Reaktion, London, 2011); Randall M. Packard, *The Making of a Tropical Disease: A Short History of Malaria* (Johns Hopkins University Press, Baltimore, 2007).

13. Packard, *Making of a Tropical Disease*; James L. A. Webb, *Humanity's Burden: A Global History of Malaria* (Cambridge University Press, Cambridge, 2009).

14. René Pleven, "Discours de clôture," in *La conférence africaine française, Brazzaville, 30 janvier–8 février 1944* (Ministère des Colonies, Paris, 1945), 67.

15. Danielle Domergue-Cloarec, "Les problèmes de santé à la conférence de Brazzaville," in Institut Charles de Gaulle and Institut d'histoire du temps présent (France) (eds.), *Brazzaville, janvier–février 1944. Aux sources de la décolonisation* (Plon, Paris, 1988), 157–69.

16. "Plan d'hygiène sociale et d'assistance médicale, recommandation de la conférence africaine française de Brazzaville," reprinted in IMTSSA, box 115, "Instruction du commissaire aux colonies, Comité français de libération nationale," 1283 Colslg/88.4, June 18, 1944.

17. Translator's note: This expression (lit., "to make blacks") was a crude but widely used call to foster African population growth.

18. IMTSSA, folder Richet, box 433, "Conférence de Brazzaville. Plan d'hygiène sociale et d'assistance médicale (version provisoire)."

19. For biographical details, see "Marcel Vaucel, 1894–1969," *Annales de l'Institut Pasteur* 119.3 (1970), 285–88; "Marcel Vaucel (1894–1969)," *Médecine Tropicale* 30.1 (1970), 1–2; A. Dubeis, "In Memoriam—Marcel Vaucel," *Annales de Société Belge de Médecine Tropicale* 50.2 (1970), 267–68; F. Blanc, "Marcel Vaucel (1894–1969)," *Bulletin de la Société de Pathologie Exotique* 64.1 (1971), 6–12.

20. Paul André Rosental, *L'intelligence démographique. Sciences et politiques des populations en France (1930–1960)* (Odile Jacob, Paris, 2003), 77–100.

21. The list of the first decrees is given in *La conférence africaine française*, 132–33. The creation of the SGHMP and SHMP has mainly been studied in the case of AOF: Danielle Domergue-Cloarec, *La santé en Côte d'Ivoire, 1905–1958*, 2 vols. (Publications de l'Université de Toulouse le Mirail, Toulouse, 1986); Jean-Paul Bado, *Les grandes endémies en Afrique, 1900–1960* (Karthala, Paris, 1996); L. Lapeyssonnie, *La médecine coloniale. Mythe et réalités* (Seghers, Paris, 1984).

22. "Instruction du commissaire aux colonies," 4.

23. AIPDak, box IPDdir9, Médecin-général Vaucel, letter to the director of the Institut Pasteur de Dakar, August 24, 1944.

24. Ministère des colonies, *Plan décennal pour le développement économique et social du Congo belge* (Éditions de Visscher, Brussels, 1949).

25. M. Kivits, "Développement des services de santé. Aperçu historique," in P. G. Janssens (ed.), *Médecine et hygiène en Afrique centrale de 1885 à nos jours* (Fondation Roi Baudouin, Brussels, 1992), 83–160; R. Mouchet, "The FOREAMI," *Transactions of the Royal Society of Tropical Medicine and Hygiene* 44.5 (1951), 483–500; Anne Cornet, *Politiques de santé et contrôle social au Rwanda 1920–1940* (Karthala, Paris, 2011).

26. This was the approach of Edgar B. Worthington in Uganda, Thomas Nash in Nigeria, and John Ford in southern Rhodesia. See Tilley, *Africa as a Living Laboratory*, 326.

27. Guillaume Lachenal, "Le médecin qui voulut être roi. Médecine coloniale et utopie au Cameroun," *Annales Histoire, Sciences Sociales* 65.1 (2010), 121–56.

28. Ibid., 147–50. The link between rubber and sleeping sickness was identified at the same time in Côte d'Ivoire, leading populations to flee. Domergue-Cloarec, *La santé en Côte d'Ivoire*, 763, 768–69, 773.

29. Farinaud, "Rapport annuel. Année 1944," 242.

30. Emanuel Lourie, L. Van Hoof, C. Henrard, and E. Peel, "Chimioprophylaxie de la maladie du sommeil par la pentamidine," *Tropical Diseases Bulletin* 44.11 (1944), 979.

31. L. Van Hoof, "Observations on Trypanosomiasis in the Belgian Congo," *Transactions of the Royal Society of Tropical Medicine and Hygiene* 40.6 (1947), 738.

32. C. C. Chesterman et al., "[Ordinary Meeting, 20th February 1947, Discussion]," *Transactions of the Royal Society of Tropical Medicine and Hygiene* 40.6 (1947), 755.

33. L. Van Hoof, C. Henrard, and E. Peel, "Chimioprophylaxie de la maladie du sommeil par la pentamidine," *Annales de Société Belge de Médecine Tropicale* 26 (1946), 381–82.

34. Farinaud, "Rapport annuel. Année 1944," 254.

35. Beaudiment, writing in IMTSSA, box 111, Médecin-colonel Farinaud, "Rapport annuel. Année 1945," 3.

36. Gaston Muraz, "Oui, l'Afrique intertropicale peut et doit guérir de la maladie du sommeil en généralisant la lomidinisation de toutes ses régions contaminées," *L'Essor Médical dans l'Union Française* 3 (1954), 15–24, 20.

37. IMTSSA, box 111, Médecin-colonel Farinaud, "Rapport annuel. Année 1946," 147.

38. The groupement was the ethnic-administrative unit on which medical screening was based; an example is the Mvélé grouping near Yaoundé.

39. Achille Mbembe, *La naissance du maquis dans le Sud Cameroun, 1920–1960* (Karthala, Paris, 1996).

40. IMTSSA, box 110, Médecin-colonel Vaisseau, "Rapport annuel. Année 1950."

41. Ibid.

42. Domergue-Cloarec, *La santé en Côte d'Ivoire*, 758.

43. Ibid., 1121–29.

44. Randall M. Packard, "The 'Healthy Reserve' and the 'Dressed Native': Discourses on Black Health and the Language of Legitimation in South Africa," *American Ethnologist* 16.4 (1989), 686–703; Megan Vaughan, *Curing Their Ills: Colonial Power and African Illness* (Polity, Cambridge, 1991).

45. Translator's note: rue Oudinot refers to the address of the Ministry of Colonies, Overseas France, in Paris.

46. Bado, *Les grandes endémies*, 370–74; Domergue-Cloarec, *La santé en Côte d'Ivoire*, 925, 1055, 1121–28.

47. Beaudiment writing in Farinaud, "Rapport annuel. Année 1946," 149.

48. IMTSSA, box 252, Commission consultative de la trypanosomiase, "Procès-verbal de la séance du 13(?) décembre 1947."

49. Bado, *Les grandes endémies*, 373; Jean-Paul Bado, "La santé et la politique en AOF à l'heure des indépendances (1939–1960)," in Charles Becker, Saliou Mbaye, and Ibrahima Thioub (eds.), *AOF. Réalités et héritages. Sociétés ouest-africaines et ordre colonial, 1895–1960* (Direction des Archives du Sénégal, Dakar, 1997), 1242–59, 1253–54.

50. L. Sanner and A. Masseguin, "Les bases légales de la médecine préventive," *Bulletin Médical de l'AOF* 11.1 (1954), 49–50.

51. Decree of June 13, 1947, *Journal Officiel du Cameroun* (1947), 875.

52. Decree 2037, June 1, 1948, *Journal Officiel du Cameroun* (1948).

53. IMTSSA, box 110, Médecin-colonel Vaisseau, "Rapport annuel. Année 1948," 97.

54. J. Le Rouzic, "Préliminaire," *Bulletin Médical de l'AOF* 6.1 (1949), 37–40, 39.

55. J.-L. McLetchie, "The Control of Sleeping Sickness in Nigeria," *Transactions of the Royal Society of Tropical Medicine and Hygiene* 41.4 (1948), 445–70.

56. This was the case in Nola, which extends into Cameroon toward Yokadouma. See G. Saleun and J. Chassain, "Essai de chimioprophylaxie de la trypanosomiase humaine en Afrique équatoriale française par la pentamidine," *Bulletin de la Société de Pathologie Exotique* 41 (1948).

57. Le Rouzic, "Préliminaire"; Domergue-Cloarec, *La santé en Côte d'Ivoire*, 1143.

58. Commission consultative de la trypanosomiase, "Procès-verbal de la séance du 13(?) décembre 1947," 8.

59. *Conférence africaine sur la tsé-tsé et la trypanosomiase. Brazzaville, 2–8 février 1948* (La Documentation Française, Toulouse, 1950). I also draw on the preparatory documents and the minutes of the conference presented by Marcel Vaucel to the Commission consultative de la trypanosomiase in 1947–48. Commission consultative de la trypanosomiase, "Procès-verbal de la séance du 13(?) décembre 1947"; IMTSSA, box 252, Commission consultative de la trypanosomiase, "Procès-verbal de la séance du 27 avril 1948."

60. Commission consultative de la trypanosomiase, "Procès-verbal de la séance du 13(?) décembre 1947," 7.

61. Ibid., 8.

62. Commission consultative de la trypanosomiase, "Procès-verbal de la séance du 27 avril 1948," 10.

63. Guillaume Lachenal, "Médecine, comparaisons et échanges inter-impériaux dans le mandat Camerounais. Une histoire croisée franco-allemande de la Mission Jamot," *Bulletin Canadien d'Histoire de la Médecine* 30.2 (2013), 23–45; Deborah Joy Neill, *Networks in Tropical Medicine: Internationalism, Colonialism, and the Rise of a Medical Specialty, 1890–1930* (Stanford University Press, Stanford, CA, 2012); Tilley, *Africa as a Living Laboratory*.

64. CAOM, Affpol/1388, Ministère de la France d'Outre-Mer, conférences diverses (rapports et correspondances), and Ministère de la France d'Outre-Mer, "Conversations franco-belges."

65. Bonnecase, *La pauvreté au Sahel*, 114.

66. Commission consultative de la trypanosomiase, "Procès-verbal de la séance du 27 avril 1948," 24.

67. McLetchie, "Control of Sleeping Sickness in Nigeria," 453.

68. L. Pinto da Fonseca, *Quimioprophylaxia pentamidinica da tripanosomiase humana em Angola* (Republica Portuguesa, Colonia de Angola, Direcçao dos Servicos de Saude e Higiene, Luanda, 1951), 18.

69. John Kent, *The Internationalization of Colonialism: Britain, France, and Black Africa, 1939–1956* (Clarendon, Oxford, 1992), 269–71.

CHAPTER 4: The Spectacle of Eradication

1. Roland Barthes, *Mythologies* (Seuil, Paris, 1957).

2. Arjun Appadurai, *Modernity at Large: Cultural Dimensions of Globalization* (University of Minnesota Press, Minneapolis, 1996), 117.

3. Florian Charvolin, *L'invention de l'environnement en France. Chroniques anthropologiques d'une institutionnalisation* (La Découverte, Paris, 2003), 123.

4. Dr. R. Beaudiment, "La lutte contre la maladie du sommeil en AOF et au Togo," *Marchés Coloniaux*, November 29, 1947.

5. These are my own estimates.

6. Arch. Spécia, box 831362B123, Spécia Saint-Fons, Correspondence (through November 1948); Direction technique, "Prévisions pour l'année 1949," January 29, 1949; Rhône-Poulenc

DUGN RTGN, July 13, 1950; Direction technique, letter to Usines Spécia, March 14, 1951; Arch. Spécia, box 124, 8313626B124, Direction commerciale, November 21, 1952.

7. On the internationalization of colonial policies in Cameroon, see Michael D. Callahan, *Mandates and Empire: The League of Nations and Africa, 1914–1931* (Sussex Academic, Brighton, England, 1999); Michael D. Callahan, *A Sacred Trust: The League of Nations and Africa, 1929–1946* (Sussex Academic, Brighton, England, 2004); Philippe Blaise Essomba, *Le Cameroun. Les rivalités d'intérêts franco-allemandes de 1919 à 1932* (Presses Universitaires de Strasbourg, Strasbourg, 2004).

8. Guillaume Lachenal, "Médecine, comparaisons et échanges inter-impériaux dans le mandat Camerounais. Une histoire croisée franco-allemande de la Mission Jamot," *Bulletin Canadien d'Histoire de la Médecine* 30.2 (2013), 23–45; Guillaume Lachenal and Bertrand Taithe, "Une généalogie missionnaire et coloniale de l'humanitaire. Le cas Aujoulat au Cameroun, 1935–1973," *Mouvement Social* 227 (2009), 45–63; Jean-Paul Bado, *Eugène Jamot, 1879–1937. Le médecin de la maladie du sommeil ou trypanosomiase* (Karthala, Paris, 2011).

9. Health spending per capita was about double in Cameroon relative to AOF and AEF. For 1927, see Rita Headrick, *Colonialism, Health and Illness in French Equatorial Africa, 1885–1935* (African Studies Association Press, Atlanta, GA, 1994), 405; for after 1945, see Richard A. Joseph, *Le mouvement nationaliste au Cameroun. Les origines sociales de l'UPC* (Karthala, Paris, 1986), 122–27.

10. IMTSSA, box 110, Médecin-colonel Vaisseau, "Rapport annuel. Année 1948," 114.

11. IMTSSA, box 110, Médecin-colonel Vaisseau, "Rapport annuel. Année 1950," section on SHMP, Nyong and Sanaga regions, n.p.

12. A. Masseguin, "La chimioprophylaxie de la trypanosomiase humaine en AOF de 1947 à 1953," *Médecine Tropicale* 13 (1953), 881–88.

13. A. Masseguin and J. Taillefer-Grimaldi, "Déclin et danger résiduel de la trypanosomiase en Afrique occidentale française," *Annales de Société Belge de Médecine Tropicale* 34–35 (1954), 671–94, 675.

14. Masseguin, "La chimioprophylaxie."

15. For example, the Compagnie minière de l'Oubangui oriental (Mining Company of Eastern Oubangui) ordered two kilograms in 1947. Arch. Spécia, box 831362B123, Spécia Saint-Fons, February 3, 1947.

16. IMTSSA, box 253, André Lotte, "La prophylaxie de la maladie du sommeil dans les zones aquatiques," 10.

17. AA, 4467/932, Dr. G. P. Lambrichts, "Note succinte sur les opérations de chimio-prophylaxie à la pentamidine sur la rive gauche du Chenal."

18. Bib. IMTA, Direction générale des services médicaux—Congo belge, "Rapport annuel 1951," 46.

19. For a retrospective overview of efforts in the Belgian Congo, see IMTSSA, box 249, Jean Demarchi, "Rapport sur la chimioprophylaxie de la trypanosomiase à *T. gambiense.*"

20. J. Burke, "Compte rendu de la chimioprophylaxie dans la région du Kasai (sous-secteur du Bas-Kwilu, FOREAMI)," *Annales de Société Belge de Médecine Tropicale* 33.1 (1953), 13–32.

21. D. Gall, "The Chemoprophylaxis of Sleeping Sickness with the Diamidines," *Annals of Tropical Medicine and Parasitology* 48.3 (1954), 242–58; J.-L. McLetchie, "The Control of Sleeping Sickness in Nigeria," *Transactions of the Royal Society of Tropical Medicine and Hygiene* 41.4 (1948), 445–70; R. D. Harding, "Mass Prophylaxis against Sleeping Sickness in Sierra Leone: Final Report," *Transactions of the Royal Society of Tropical Medicine and Hygiene* 43 (1950), 503–12.

22. L. Pinto da Fonseca, *Quimioprophylaxia pentamidinica da tripanosomiase humana em Angola* (Republica Portuguesa, Colonia de Angola, Direcçao dos Servicos de Saude e Higiene, Luanda, 1951).

23. Jorge Varanda, "Crossing Colonies and Empires: The Health Services of the Diamond Company of Angola," in Anne Digby, Ernst Waltraud, and Projit B. Muhkarji (eds.), *Crossing Colonial Historiographies: Histories of Colonial and Indigenous Medicines in Transnational Perspective* (Cambridge Scholars Publishing, Cambridge, 2010), 165–84.

24. Gall, "Chemoprophylaxis."

25. W. Eraerts, "La propamidine comme préventif dans deux foyers de trypanosomiase humaine au Congo belge," *Annales de Société Belge de Médecine Tropicale* 27 (1947), 221.

26. B. B. Waddy, "Chemioprophylaxis of Human Trypanosomiasis," in H. W. Mulligan and W. H. Potts (eds.), *The African Trypanosomiases* (Allen and Unwin, London, 1970), 711–25, 723–24.

27. For example, see Service général autonome de la maladie du sommeil, *Organisation du Service de prophylaxie et de traitement de la maladie du sommeil en AOF et au Togo* (Imprimerie Polyglotte Africaine, Maison-Carrée, Algeria), 1942.

28. Rapport annuel du gouvernement français sur l'administration sous mandat des territoires du Cameroun pour l'année 1931 (Imprimerie Générale Lahire, Paris, 1932), 87.

29. The standardization of treatment was debated in the 1930s. See Gaston Muraz, "À propos de la 'cure standard' appliquée, en Afrique équatoriale française, aux trypanosomés," *Bulletin de la Société de Pathologie Exotique* 23 (1930), 917–22; Gaston Muraz, "Le traitement standard de la maladie du sommeil," *Bulletin de la Société de Pathologie Exotique* 24.7 (1931), 530–34; Gaston Muraz, "Quelques derniers mots au sujet de la 'cure standard' de la maladie du sommeil," *Bulletin de la Société de Pathologie Exotique* 25.1 (1932), 39–43; Headrick, *Colonialism, Health and Illness*, 331–32.

30. On Céline, Fordism, and standardized medicine, see Philippe Roussin, *Misère de la littérature, terreur de l'histoire. Céline et la littérature contemporaine* (Gallimard, Paris, 2005), 90–110.

31. IMTSSA, box 108, "Rapport annuel à l'ONU [Organisation des nations unies] pour l'année 1952. Santé publique."

32. The issue was debated as early as 1947 by English experimenters, notably C. C. Chesterman et al., "[Ordinary Meeting, 20th February 1947, Discussion]," *Transactions of the Royal Society of Tropical Medicine and Hygiene* 40.6 (1947), 755–61.

33. AA, 1064/Missions experts, Dr. R. Haddad, "Conseils en vue d'un contrôle permanent de la trypanosomiase humaine au Soudan," 1955.

34. IMTSSA, box 253, André Lotte, "Rapport complémentaire sur les accidents septiques observés dans le secteur IV," March 4, 1953, appendix 1:3.

35. F. Gauthier, Lutte contre la trypanosomiase et la lèpre en Afrique 1953–1960. Mission d'une équipe médicale mobile de prospection du Service général d'hygiène et de prophylaxie (Éditions des Écrivains, Paris, 2000), 104.

36. Cited in Jacques Pierre Ziegler, "Contribution à l'étude de la chimioprophylaxie de la maladie du sommeil, no. 313," thesis for doctorate in medicine, Faculté de médecine de Paris, 1948, 129.

37. Lotte, "Rapport complémentaire,"appendix 1:3.

38. G. Pille, "Considérations pharmacologiques sur les diamidines et leur utilisation dans la trypanosomiase," *Médecine Tropicale* 13 (1953), 859–69, 864.

39. Pentamidine (MB 800) and Lomidine (2512 RP) were initially formulated in dihydrochloride form. English Pentamidine was later reformulated as a diisethionate salt. Used in 1946–47 in the French Empire, MB 800 was then replaced after 1948 by its French version —Lomidine—which now used a different base, dimesilate. But Lomidine, which was sent to the colonies in powder form, was much less soluble than MB 800; it was not possible, in the field, to obtain solutions with concentrations higher than 2 percent (versus 4 percent with the May & Baker powder). For a standard dose of 4 milligrams per kilogram, the use of Lo-

midine thus meant that an individual would need to be injected with 15 cubic centimeters of solution (versus 5–7 cubic centimeters with Pentamidine). For this reason, the dimesilate powder was quickly abandoned, and Lomidine was formulated for the mass campaigns as either industrially prepared ampules of 4 percent solution or as diisethionate powder. Ziegler, "Contribution," 82.

40. Ziegler, "Contribution," 85–90; Demarchi, "Rapport sur la chimioprophylaxie."

41. Jorge Varanda, pers. comm.

42. Masseguin, "La chimioprophylaxie."

43. IMTSSA, box 103, R. Beaudiment, "Étude sur la chimioprophylaxie, étude sur les résultats du traitement par l'Arsobal, ou Mel B," 1–2; and R. Beaudiment and R. Zozol, "Expérimentation clinique de l'effet tampon du Moranyl sur la Lomidine, en vue de son application à la prophylaxie de masse et éventuellement au traitement de la période lymphatico-sanguine," in "Rapport annuel 1952 du BPITT," ISCTR (52), 28. The method of combining Lomidine and Moranyl was also tested in French West Africa; see A. Masseguin, M. Causse, and M. Ricosse, "Note préliminaire sur l'association Lomidine-Moranyl, dans la prévention de la maladie du sommeil," *Bulletin de la Société de Pathologie Exotique* 48.1 (1955), 36–37.

44. Demarchi, "Rapport sur la chimioprophylaxie," 5.

45. Interview by author with Jean Meno, Yaoundé, 2005.

46. André Lotte, "Essai de codification de la prophylaxie chimique de la maladie du sommeil," *Médecine Tropicale* 13 (1953), 889–948, 919.

47. Ibid.

48. André Lotte, "Enseignements de quatre années de chimioprophylaxie en AEF," *Médecine Tropicale* 11.5 (1951), 737–66.

49. Lotte invented the prophylactic K coefficient, calculated from the curb (exponential decrease) of the index of circulating virus (IVC, the prevalence index) during Lomidinization: $IVC(t) = IVC_0 \cdot e^{-Kt}$. The greater the K coefficient, the more an epidemic focus was sensitive to chemoprophylaxis. See Lotte, "Essai de codification." Lotte's classification was also used by some anglophone authors and in manuals such as Marcel Vaucel's *Médecine tropicale*, 2nd ed. (Flammarion, Paris, 1959).

50. R. Beaudiment and P. Leproux, "Incidence de la lomidinisation sur la régression de la trypanosomiase au Cameroun français," *Médecine Tropicale* 13 (1953), 949–54, 951.

51. Lotte, "Essai de codification," 918.

52. Christophe Bonneuil, "Development as Experiment," *Osiris* 14 (2001), 258–81.

53. IMTSSA, box 103, André Lotte, "Enseignements de quatre années de propylaxie en AEF," 24.

54. For a calculation of a campaign's costs in Angola, for example, see Pinto da Fonseca, *Quimioprophylaxia.*

55. IMTSSA, Fonds Richet, box 428, Chemise SGAMS, Dr. Kernevez, "SGHMP. Instructions au sujet de l'emploi des diamidines dans la chimioprophylaxie de la trypanosomiase humaine," 6.

56. Lotte, "Essai de codification," 920.

57. Masseguin, "La chimioprophylaxie," 886.

58. IMTSSA, box 253, Médecin-colonel Masseguin, "Manuscrit typographié. La chimioprophylaxie de la trypanosomiase humaine en AOF de 1947 à 1953," 8.

59. Jean-François Bayart, Le gouvernement du monde. Une critique politique de la globalisation (Fayard, Paris, 2004), 197–250.

60. Ziegler, "Contribution," 130. Jacques Pierre Ziegler (b. 1923) graduated from the Institut de médecine coloniale (Colonial Medical Institute) of the Faculty of Medicine of Paris but was not a member of the colonial corps. After a career in several African countries working for

the SGHMP, the French cooperation with the WHO, Jacques Pierre Ziegler retired in Switzerland. He was not able to answer my questions for health reasons.

61. Jean Dutertre, "Jean-Marc et la trypano," perso.orange.fr/jdtr/Jeanmarc.htm, accessed July 2, 2006.

62. Lapeyssonnie, "Mais qu'est-ce qui faisait donc courir le Docteur Gambadus?" in Collectif (ed.), *Sillages et feux de brousse*, vol. 2 (Association des Anciens Élèves de l'École du Service de Santé des Armées de Bordeaux, Paris, 1992), 124–31, 15–16.

63. IMTSSA, box 253, Anonymous, "Applications de la chimioprophylaxie à la trypanosomiase humaine en AEF," 26; box 103, Anonymous, "Les grandes endémies et épidémies. Trypanosomiase," 9.

64. Vaisseau, "Rapport annuel. Année 1950," section on SHMP, Nyong, and Sanaga, n.p.

65. Kernevez, "SGHMP. Instructions," 5.

66. André Lotte, "Historique du foyer de trypanosomiase de Nola," *Bulletin de la Société de Pathologie Exotique* 46.3 (1953), 374–86, 381.

67. ANY, APA 10 876, Médecin-colonel Vaisseau, "Rapport annuel. Année 1951," 14.

68. C. Hollins et al., "[Ordinary Meeting, 11th December 1947, Discussion]," *Transactions of the Royal Society of Tropical Medicine and Hygiene* 41.4 (1948), 471–80, 475.

69. L. Pinto da Fonseca, *Chimioprophylaxie par la pentamidine de la trypanosomiase humaine en Angola* (République Portugaise, Colonie d'Angola, Direction des Services de Santé et Hygiène, Luanda, 1951), in Pinto da Fonseca, *Quimioprophylaxia*. French translation by Jacques Pépin, illegible page number.

70. P. Le Gac and Jacques Pierre Ziegler, "La trypanosomiase en Oubangui-Chari, le foyer de l'Ouham. Sa prophylaxie par la lomidine," *Bulletin de la Société de Pathologie Exotique* 45.2 (1952), 235–42.

71. "Les progrès dans la lutte contre la maladie du sommeil," *France d'Outre-Mer Bulletin d'Information* (1949), 6, ufdc.ufl.edu/?b=UF00080165&v=00006, accessed September 10, 2013.

72. H. Kernevez and J. Chassain, "Note sur les résultats obtenus en Afrique équatoriale française par l'emploi des diamidines dans la chimioprophylaxie de la trypanosomiase humaine (période de 1946 à 1949)," *Bulletin de la Société de Pathologie Exotique* 44.5–6 (1951), 337–43, 337.

73. J. Diallo, "Résultats de la chimioprophylaxie par les diamidines dans le secteur spécial no. 3, à Guéckédou-Kissidougou (Guinée)," *Bulletin de la Société de Pathologie Exotique* 44.1–2 (1951), 93–103, 93.

74. P. Le Gac, "La trypanosomiase en Oubangui-Chari, le foyer de Nola. Sa chimioprophylaxie par la pentamidine et la lomidine," *Bulletin de la Société de Pathologie Exotique* 44.7–8 (1951), 488–94, 494.

75. H. Jonchère, "Chimioprophylaxie de la trypanosomiase humaine en AOF," *Bulletin de la Société de Pathologie Exotique* 44.1–2 (1951), 83–93, 92.

76. IMTSSA, box 253, Anonymous, "Vue d'ensemble sur la trypanosomiase en AOF en 1952."

77. Anonymous, "Les grandes endémies et épidémies," 9.

78. Pinto da Fonseca, *Quimioprophylaxia*, 17, translated by Mariana Broglia de Moura.

79. Ibid., 18.

80. Ibid.

81. Anonymous, "Applications de la chimioprophylaxie," 23.

82. J. H. Raynal, "Sur la trypanosomiase humaine africaine et sa prophylaxie," *Médecine Tropicale* 13 (1953), 793–98, 795.

83. Experimenting on soldiers interned in the military psychiatric hospital of Marseille—mostly African soldiers evacuated from Indochina—the inoculation of trypanosomes had

promising effects in some psychiatric conditions, such as schizophrenia, sometimes even leading to complete recovery. P. Gallais, "La trypanosomiase d'inoculation expérimentale. Réflexions neurologiques et philosophie d'un essai thérapeutique," *Médecine Tropicale* 13 (1953), 799–806.

84. Raynal, "Sur la trypanosomiase humaine africaine et sa prophylaxie," 796.

85. Anonymous, "Applications de la chimioprophylaxie," 26.

86. Ziegler, "Contribution"; J. Anquez, "Chimioprophylaxie de la maladie du sommeil par la pentamidine ou lomidine, no. 588," thesis for doctorate in medicine, Faculty of Medicine, Paris, 1949.

87. G. Fesquet, "Les diamidines aromatiques dans la trypanosomiase," *Médecine Tropicale* 8.3 (1948), 348–50.

88. BIUP, Dossier biographique Léon Launoy, Cote D LAU 2, Anonymous, "Léon Launoy 1876–1971."

89. Gaston Muraz, "Oui, l'Afrique intertropicale peut et doit guérir de la maladie du sommeil en généralisant la lomidinisation de toutes ses régions contaminées," *L'Essor Médical dans l'Union Française* 3 (1954), 23, emphasis in original. Muraz was notably the author of two collections of poems and photographs: *Satyres illustrées de l'Afrique noire* (Éditions du Comité de Documentation et de Propagande de l'Afrique Noire Française, Paris, 1947); and *Sous le grand soleil, chez les primitifs. Images d'Afrique équatoriale* (Paul Brodard, Coulommiers, France, 1923).

90. Gaston Muraz, "L'éradication de la maladie du sommeil par la lomidinisation," *L'Essor Médical dans l'Union Française* 4 (1954), 45–55, 54, emphasis in original.

91. Gaston Muraz, "Des très larges mesures de chimioprophylaxie par injections intramusculaires de diamidines aromatiques (lomidine) mises en œuvre depuis plusieurs années déjà et tendant à l'éradication de la maladie du sommeil dans les territoires de l'Afrique noire française (AOF, AEF, Cameroun et Togo sous mandat), contaminés de cette endémie," *Bulletin de l'Académie Nationale de Médecine* 138.33–35 (1954), 617.

92. Gall, "Chemoprophylaxis," 242.

93. AA, 4485/1063, article sent by the Belgian Congo Trade Mission in New York (*New York Herald Tribune*, January 19, 1948).

94. L. Pinto da Fonseca, "The Cartographic Representation of Areas Surveyed after a First Treatment with Pentamidine," paper presented at the fourth meeting of the International Scientific Committee for Trypanosomiasis Research, Lourenço Marques, September 25–30, 1952. See also BPITT, Permanent Inter-African Bureau for Tsetse and Trypanosomiasis, Léopoldville, 1952, 195.

CHAPTER 5. Lomidine, the Individual, and Race

1. L. Aujoulat, "Le rôle social du médecin dans la France d'Outre-Mer," *Semaine des Hôpitaux* 27.11 (1951), 488–89, 488.

2. On accidents as revealing of nonhuman agency, see Bruno Latour, *Changer de société, refaire de la sociologie* (La Découverte, Paris, 2006).

3. Léon Launoy, "Sur le comportement du rat après une ou plusieurs de *T. gambiense* pratiquées sous le couvert de doses variables de diméthane sulfontate du diamidinophénoxypentane," *Médecine Tropicale* 13 (1953), 870–80.

4. J. H. Raynal, "Sur la trypanosomiase humaine africaine et sa prophylaxie," *Médecine Tropicale* 13 (1953), 793–98, 797.

5. Léon Launoy in *Bulletin des Sciences Pharmacologiques* 37 (1930), 105, quoted in Jacques Pierre Ziegler, "Contribution à l'étude de la chimioprophylaxie de la maladie du sommeil, no. 313," thesis for doctorate in medicine, Faculté de médecine de Paris, 1948, 614.

6. Christoph Gradmann, "Robert Koch and the Invention of the Carrier State: Tropical

Medicine, Veterinary Infections and Epidemiology around 1900," *Studies in History and Philosophy of Biological and Biomedical Sciences* 41 (2010), 232–40.

7. Echoes of contemporary HIV policies of treatment-as-prevention are not coincidental. See Guillaume Lachenal, "A Genealogy of 'Treatment-as-Prevention,'" in Tamara Giles-Vernick and James L. A. Webb (eds.), *Global Health Histories in Africa* (Ohio University Press, Athens, 2013), 70–91.

8. Léon Lapeyssonnie, *Toubib des tropiques* (Robert Laffont, Paris, 1982), 96.

9. For example, in Algeria, see E. Collignon, "Sur le coût de la quinisation des réservoirs de virus paludéen en Algérie," *Bulletin de la Société de Pathologie Exotique* 29 (1936), 1090–93; Edmond Sergent, "La quininisation en Algérie," *Bulletin de la Société de Pathologie Exotique* 1 (1908), 534–36.

10. Pierre Louis Émile Millous, "Le traitement de la maladie du sommeil au Cameroun," *Annales de Médecine et de Pharmacie Coloniales* 34 (1936), 966–95, 967.

11. Ziegler, "Contribution à l'étude de la chimioprophylaxie de la maladie du sommeil," 114.

12. *Conférence africaine sur la tsé-tsé et la trypanosomiase. Brazzaville, 2–8 février 1948* (La Documentation Française, Toulouse, 1950), 239–40.

13. André Lotte, "Essai de codification de la prophylaxie chimique de la maladie du sommeil," *Médecine Tropicale* 13 (1953), 908.

14. R. D. Harding, "Mass Prophylaxis against Sleeping Sickness in Sierra Leone: Final Report," *Transactions of the Royal Society of Tropical Medicine and Hygiene* 43 (1950), 503–12.

15. G. Pille, "Considérations pharmacologiques sur les diamidines et leur utilisation dans la trypanosomiase," *Médecine Tropicale* 13 (1953), 859–69.

16. *Conférence africaine sur la tsé-tsé et la trypanosomiase*, 217–19.

17. Ibid., 21.

18. Ibid.

19. Ibid.

20. IMTSSA, box 103, "Enquête sur les glossines effectuée dans la subdivision de Yokadouma, 1949." See also box 249, Jean Demarchi, "Rapport sur la chimioprophylaxie de la trypanosomiase à *T. gambiense*," 27.

21. Pille, "Considérations pharmacologiques," 859.

22. Lotte, "Essai de codification," 911.

23. Ibid., 921.

24. Ibid., 918.

25. A. Masseguin, "La chimioprophylaxie de la trypanosomiase humaine en AOF de 1947 à 1953," *Médecine Tropicale* 13 (1953), 887.

26. For example, in the case of quininization, see Edmond Sergent et al., "De l'emploi de la quinine contre le paludisme," *Bulletin de la Société de Pathologie Exotique* 18 (1925), 28–36.

27. R. D. Harding and M. P. Hutchinson, "Sleeping Sickness of an Unusual Type in Sierra Leone and Its Attempted Control," *Transactions of the Royal Society of Tropical Medicine and Hygiene* 41.4 (1948), 481–512, 503.

28. Lotte, "Essai de codification," 909.

29. Ibid., 906.

30. Ibid., 907.

31. Jacques Pierre Ziegler, "Rapport annuel du secteur XII," cited ibid., 907–8.

32. "Rapport du médecin-chef du secteur 2, Dolisie, 1949," cited ibid., 908.

33. Sloan Mahone, "The Psychology of Rebellion: Colonial Medical Responses to Dissent in British East Africa," *Journal of African History* 47.2 (2006), 241–58.

34. J. Burke, "Compte rendu de la chimioprophylaxie dans la région du Kasai (sous-secteur du Bas-Kwilu, FOREAMI)," *Annales de Société Belge de Médecine Tropicale* 33.1 (1953), 13–32.

35. Gaston Muraz, "Oui, l'Afrique intertropicale peut et doit guérir de la maladie du sommeil en généralisant la lomidinisation de toutes ses régions contaminées," *L'Essor Médical dans l'Union Française* 3 (1954), 24.

36. IMTSSA, box 253, Anonymous, "Applications de la chimioprophylaxie à la trypanosomiase humaine en AEF," 26.

37. IMTSSA, Fonds Richet, box 428, Médecin-colonel Gaston Muraz, "Note de service du 25 octobre 1941." For an example of a dramatic accident that occurred in Guinea in 1941, see IMTSSA, Fonds Richet, box 433, Médecin-commandant Richet, "Rapport au médecin-colonel Gaston Muraz, 22 décembre 1941," no. 88 TR.

38. Médecin-colonel Richet, "Quelques considérations sur la chimio-prophylaxie de la trypanosomiase humaine en A.E.F.," in *International Scientific Committee for Trypanosomiasis Research: Fifth Meeting, Held at Pretoria 13th to 17th September, 1954* (BPITT, Léopoldville, 1954), 72–84, 77.

39. For example, a systematic inquiry into cases of post-Lomidinization hypoglycemia was mandated by Richet in 1955. See IMTSSA, Fonds Richet, box 428.

40. IMTSSA, box 253, R. Beaudiment, L. Cauvin, and Ph. Leproux, "Accidents de lomidinisation au Cameroun français. Leur thérapeutique et leur prévention [expérimentation du 4891 RP]."

41. "Vagosympathetic" refers here to the sudden activation of the sympathetic nervous system (which leads to hypotensive effects) following a reflex regulatory action involving the vagus nerve. This phenomenon is better known as a "vagal episode."

42. Beaudiment, Cauvin, and Leproux, "Accidents de lomidinisation."

43. Ibid.

44. Ibid.

45. Ibid.

46. Ziegler, "Contribution," 29.

47. L. Pinto da Fonseca, "The Cartographic Representation of Areas Surveyed after a First Treatment with Pentamidine," paper presented at the fourth meeting of the International Scientific Committee for Trypanosomiasis Research, Lourenço-Marques, September 25–30, 1952, 17.

48. Noémi Tousignant, "Trypanosomes, Toxicity and Resistance: The Politics of Mass Therapy in French Colonial Africa," *Social History of Medicine* 25.3 (2012), 625–43.

49. Translator's note: The term used in French was *blanchir* (lit., "to bleach"), meaning to sanitize or sterilize.

50. A. Fain in *Rec. Trav. Sc. Med. Congo Belge* (1942), 137, cited in Ziegler, "Contribution," 71.

51. H. Lester, "Further Progress in the Control of Sleeping Sickness in Nigeria," *Transactions of the Royal Society of Tropical Medicine and Hygiene* 38.6 (1945), 425–44, 436.

52. D. Gall, "The Chemoprophylaxis of Sleeping Sickness with the Diamidines," *Annals of Tropical Medicine and Parasitology* 48.3 (1954), 254.

53. For an example of such rhetoric, see IMTSSA, box 356, "Compte-rendu sur le groupe de travail de la CCTA, Léopoldville," September 25,1954.

54. A. J. Duggan, cited in J. Burke, "Historique de la lutte contre la maladie du sommeil au Congo," *Annales de Société Belge de Médecine Tropicale* 51.4–6 (1971), 465–77, 481.

55. Lotte, "Essai de codification," 919.

56. H. Jonchère, "Chimioprophylaxie de la trypanosomiase humaine en AOF," *Bulletin de la Société de Pathologie Exotique* 44.1–2 (1951), 88, emphasis in original.

57. "Une maladie qui disparaît. La maladie du sommeil," *Hygiène et Alimentation au Cameroun* (July 1, 1953), 19, 14.

58. Marcel Vaucel, *Médecine tropicale*, 2nd ed. (Flammarion, Paris, 1959), 568.

59. IMTSSA, Fonds Richet, box 428, Chemise SGAMS, Dr. Kernevez, "SGHMP. Instructions au sujet de l'emploi des diamidines dans la chimioprophylaxie de la trypanosomiase humaine."

60. AIPDak, box IPDDir1, Noël Bernard, letter to Dr. Camille Durieux, director of the Institut Pasteur de l'AOF, September 26, 1950.

61. Vaucel, *Médecine tropicale*, 566.

62. L. Nodenot, "Note sur une infection accidentelle avec une souche de *Trypanosoma gambiense*," *Bulletin de la Société de Pathologie Exotique* 42 (1949), 16–18.

63. Arch. Spécia, box 124, 8313626B124, Direction technique, letter to Spécia Saint-Fons, May 18, 1954, no. 2768.

64. Personal communication with the author, 2011.

65. Arch. Spécia, box 831362B123, Spécia, "Projet de prospectus."

CHAPTER 6: Good Citizens and Bad Brothers

1. IMTSSA, box 110, Médecin-colonel Vaisseau, "Rapport annuel. Année 1947," 112.

2. Médecin-colonel Richet, "Quelques considérations sur la chimio-prophylaxie de la trypanosomiase humaine en A.E.F.," in *International Scientific Committee for Trypanosomiasis Research: Fifth Meeting, Held at Pretoria 13th to 17th September, 1954* (BPITT, Léopoldville, 1954), 72–84, 83.

3. Translator's note: Some neutral pronouns in the original text have been translated into English as masculine in this chapter as a reflection of common usage at the time, in which an anonymous individual was generally referred to as masculine.

4. This (ableist) term was used by Fred Cooper and Jane Burbank to describe the colonialism of the (French) Fourth Republic (1946–58). See Burbank and Cooper, *Empires in World History: Power and the Politics of Difference* (Princeton University Press, Princeton, NJ, 2010), 422.

5. Dr. M. Peltier, "Éducation hygiénique des populations indigènes," *Annales d'Hygiène et de Médecine Coloniales* 33 (1935), 969–76.

6. Romain Bertrand, *État colonial, noblesse et nationalisme à Java* (Karthala, Paris, 2005), 388–99; Warwick Anderson, *Colonial Pathologies: American Tropical Medicine, Race and Hygiene in the Philippines* (Duke University Press, Durham, NC, 2006), 180–206.

7. Armelle Mabon, *L'action sociale coloniale. L'exemple de l'Afrique occidentale française du Front populaire à la veille des indépendances* (L'Harmattan, Paris, 2000); Nancy Rose Hunt, "Domesticity and Colonialism in Belgian Africa: Usumbura's Foyer Social, 1946–1960," *Signs* 15.3 (1990), 447–74.

8. Frederick Cooper, *Decolonization and African Society: The Labor Question in French and British Africa* (Cambridge University Press, Cambridge, 1996), 15.

9. Bertrand, *État colonial, noblesse et nationalisme à Java*, 662.

10. *Rapport annuel du gouvernement français à l'Assemblée générale des Nations unies sur l'administration du Cameroun placé sous la tutelle de la France: 1948* (Lavauzelle, Paris, 1949), 119.

11. Guillaume Lachenal and Bertrand Taithe, "Une généalogie missionaire et coloniale de l'humanitaire. Le cas Aujoulat au Cameroun, 1935–1973," *Mouvement Social* 227 (2009), 45–63.

12. Bertrand, *État colonial, noblesse et nationalisme à Java*, 456.

13. Pauline Kuziak, "Instrumentalized Rationality, Cross-Cultural Mediators, and Civil Epistemologies of Late Colonialism," *Social Studies of Science* 40.6 (2010), 871–902; Hunt, "Domesticity and Colonialism"; F. Herman and J. Courtejoie, "Éducation sanitaire," in P. G. Janssens (ed.), *Médecine et hygiène en Afrique centrale de 1885 à nos jours* (Fondation Roi Baudouin, Brussels, 1992), 549–60, 552.

14. *Rapport annuel du gouvernement français à l'Assemblée générale des Nations unies sur l'administration du Cameroun placé sous la tutelle de la France: 1952* (Lavauzelle, Paris, 1953), 228–29.

15. *Rapport annuel du gouvernement français à l'Assemblée générale des Nations unies sur l'administration du Cameroun placé sous la tutelle de la France: 1950* (Lavauzelle, Paris, 1951), 250.

16. Megan Vaughan, *Curing Their Ills: Colonial Power and African Illness* (Polity, Cambridge, 1991), 180–99; Timothy Burke, "'Our Mosquitoes Are Not So Big': Images and Modernity in Zimbabwe," in P. Landau and D. Kaspin (eds.), *Images and Empires: Visuality in Colonial and Postcolonial Africa* (University of California Press, Berkeley, 2002), 41–55.

17. Eric A. Stein, "Colonial Theatres of Proof: Representation and Laughter in 1930s Rockefeller Foundation Hygiene Cinema in Java," *Health and History* 8.2 (2006), 14–44.

18. Vinh-Kim Nguyen, *The Republic of Therapy: Triage and Sovereignty in West Africa's Time of AIDS* (Duke University Press, Durham, NC, 2010).

19. *Hygiène et Alimentation au Cameroun* 1 (July 1, 1948), back cover.

20. Anonymous, "Les méfaits de l'alcoolisme," *Hygiène et Alimentation au Cameroun* 18 (April 1, 1953), 11.

21. Luc Berlivet, "Une biopolitique de l'éducation pour la santé. La fabrique des campagnes de prévention," in Didier Fassin and Dominique Memmi (eds.), *Le gouvernement des corps* (Éditions de l'EHESS, Paris, 2004), 37–75.

22. *Hygiène et Alimentation au Cameroun*, vols. 1–20 (1948–53).

23. *Hygiène et Alimentation au Cameroun* 18 (April 1953), 1.

24. L. Pinto da Fonseca, *Quimioprophylaxia pentamidinica da tripanosomiase humana em Angola* (Republica Portuguesa, Colonia de Angola, Direcçao dos Servicos de Saude e Higiene, Luanda, 1951), 17–19.

25. Ibid., 18.

26. SHMP, "Trypanosomiase et Lomidine," *Hygiène et Alimentation au Cameroun* 16 (October 1, 1952), 5.

27. Ibid.

28. IMTSSA, box 110, Médecin-colonel Vaisseau, "Rapport annuel. Année 1950," SHMP, region Haut-Nyong, n.p.

29. Arch. Spécia, box 124, 8313626B124, Dr. Ziegler, letter to Dr. de Marqueissac, reproduced in "Lettre de la Direction technique, no. 2703," June 25, 1953.

30. Priscilla Wald, *Contagious: Cultures, Carriers, and the Outbreak Narrative* (Duke University Press, Durham, NC, 2008).

31. Paul Weindling, *Epidemics and Genocide in Eastern Europe, 1890–1945* (Oxford University Press, Oxford, 2000).

32. André Lotte, "Essai de codification de la prophylaxie chimique de la maladie du sommeil," *Médecine Tropicale* 13 (1953), 910.

33. "Heads of household will be responsible for their families, the husband of the wife and both of their children; *regedores* and *sobetas* [customary chiefs] will be responsible for all, including those who have no relatives and of their own guests." Quoted in Pinto da Fonseca, *Quimioprophylaxia*, 19.

34. Berlivet, "Une biopolitique."

35. "CAOM, Affpol 2688, Ministre des colonies, "Rapport au président de la république. Condamnation à mort Biyong N'dengue"; and Ministre des colonies, "Rapport au président de la république. Recours en grâce du nommé N'Gote Bongo, condamné à mort."

36. Mahmood Mamdani, *Citizen and Subject: Contemporary Africa and the Legacy of Late Colonialism* (Princeton University Press, Princeton, NJ, 1996).

37. Arch. CSE, 2D54 A, "Résumé de journaux de communautés, fascicule X (Yokadouma)," and Mission de Yokadouma, "Résumé du journal," November 1, 1947, 43.

38. Danielle Domergue-Cloarec, *La santé en Côte d'Ivoire, 1905–1958*, 2 vols. (Publications de l'Université de Toulouse le Mirail, Toulouse, 1986), 1113.

39. Ibid., 1128.

40. "Résumé de journaux de communautés," and Mission de Yokadouma, "Résumé du journal," 47.

41. Tamara Giles-Vernick, *Cutting the Vines of the Past: Environmental Histories of the Central African Rain Forest* (University Press of Virginia, Charlottesville, 2002), 106.

42. Médecin-colonel Nodenot, reply to Service des grandes épidémies de l'AOF, reproduced in IMTSSA, box 249, Jean Demarchi, "Rapport sur la chimioprophylaxie de la trypanosomiase à *T. gambiense.*"

43. IMTSSA, Fonds Richet, box 433, Médecin-commandant Richet, "Compte rendu no 88/TR de l'inspection du secteur spécial no. 29 (Labé) faite, les 24–25–26 novembre 1941, par le médecin-commandant adjoint au chef du Service général de la maladie du sommeil en AOF et au Togo."

44. Maxime Lamotte, interview with author, Paris, 2003.

45. Domergue-Cloarec, *La santé en Côte d'Ivoire*, 153–55.

46. Jacques Ferret, *Les cendres du Manengouba* (L'Harmattan, Paris, 1996), 176–79.

47. Note the confusion (which was very common) between Lomidinization and vaccination.

48. Ferret, *Les cendres du Manengouba*, 179.

49. Ibid., 176.

50. Ibid., 179.

51. ANY, APA 10 876, Médecin-colonel Vaisseau, "Rapport annuel. Année 1951," section on SHMP, Yaoundé, and Tribu Bané, n.p.

52. Ferret, *Cendres du Manengouba*, 179.

53. Thomas Deltombe, Manuel Domergue, and Jacob Tatsitsa, *Kamerun! Une guerre cachée aux origines de la Françafrique, 1948–1971* (La Découverte, Paris, 2011), 273–74.

CHAPTER 7: Yokadouma, Cameroon, November–December 1954

1. ANY, 3 AC 1871, "Télégramme officiel de région Yokadouma pour Santé publique Yaoundé," no. 195/TO/RFN, November 15, 1954.

2. Luc Boltanski and Ève Chiapello, *Le nouvel esprit du capitalisme* (Gallimard, Paris, 1999), 73–80.

3. ANY, 3 AC 1871, Christol, "Rapport de l'inspecteur des Affaires administratives du centre. Décès à la suite de la campagne de lomidinisation du GM 15 du SHMP à Yokadouma du 14 au 17 novembre," November 22, 1954, 1.

4. IMTSSA, box 108, "Rapport annuel à l'ONU pour l'année 1953. Santé publique"; IMTSSA, box 108, "Rapport annuel à l'ONU pour l'année 1954. Santé publique," 95.

5. André Lotte, "Historique du foyer de trypanosomiase de Nola," *Bulletin de la Société de Pathologie Exotique* 46.3 (1953), 374–86.

6. Christol, "Rapport de l'inspecteur des Affaires administratives du centre," 1.

7. Arch. CSE, 2J1.10.13, Yaoundé file, correspondence 1934–35, Monsignor Graffin, letter to Monsignor (Hunsec?), April 5, 1935.

8. IMTSSA, box 110, Médecin-colonel Vaisseau, "Rapport annuel. Année 1950," section on SHMP, Lom, and Kadei, n.p.

9. ANY, 3 AC 1871, Direction des affaires administratives et politiques, "Rapport confidentiel du haut-commissaire au Ministre de la France d'Outre-Mer. Accidents survenus au cours campagne lomidinisation région Boumba-Ngoko," December 31, 1954, 1.

10. ANY, 3 AC 1871, Gilbrin, "Rapport du chef de région de la Boumba-Ngoko à M. le haut-commissaire de la République française au Cameroun. Accidents mortels suite passage GMT 15," November 19, 1954.

11. African doctor (*médecin africain*) was the official title given to doctors trained at the School of Medicine of Dakar.

12. Christol, "Rapport de l'inspecteur," 3.

13. Gilbrin, "Rapport du chef de région," 4.

14. Christol, "Rapport de l'inspecteur," 3.

15. Gilbrin, "Rapport du chef de région," 4.

16. ANY, 3 AC 1871, "Extrait du rapport politique mensuel, région Boumba-Ngoko," November 1954; Gilbrin, "Rapport du chef de région," 4.

17. ANY, 3 AC 1871, Assemblée territoriale du Cameroun, "Session extraordinaire d'octobre 1954. PV de la séance plénière du 18 novembre 1954," 12.

18. Gilbrin, "Rapport du chef de région," 4.

19. ANY, 3 AC 1871, "Télégramme officiel chiffré de région Yokadouma pour haut-commissaire de la RF au Cameroun," November 19, 1954.

20. ANY, 3 AC 1871, "Télégramme officiel chiffré de région Yokadouma pour haut-commissaire de la RF au Cameroun, novembre 14 à 18," November 18, 1954.

21. These categories were defined for triage purposes by Dr. Constant. The description given for the "critical" condition was "edema spreading beyond the gluteal area, reaching the thighs and in some cases the abdominal wall and the genital organs; crepitus, blistering, general phenomena characteristic of toxemia. Upon incision emission of nonfetid gas." "Serious" cases were described as having "voluminous edema of the gluteal area with crepitus and discrete general phenomena"; "less serious" was "induration with localized inflammatory response," while "slight" cases had "simple induration at the site of injection." ANY, 3 AC 1871, Médecin-lieutenant-colonel Cauvin, "Rapport du chef du Service d'hygiène mobile et de prophylaxie à monsieur le directeur des services de la Santé publique au Cameroun," November 24, 1954, 3.

22. The classic reference on this point is Edward W. Said, *Culture and Imperialism* (Knopf, New York, 1993), vii.

23. Gilbrin, "Rapport du chef de région," 7; Christol, "Rapport de l'inspecteur," 6; Cauvin, "Rapport du chef," 9 and 2; ANY, 3 AC 1871, Capitaine Jardin, "Compte rendu du commandant de section de gendarmerie à Monsieur le haut-commissaire de la République française au Cameroun et à Monsieur le procureur général," November 26, 1954, 2.

24. "Extrait du rapport politique mensuel."

25. *Bacillus perfringens* has since been reclassified as *Clostridium perfringens*. Gas gangrene was a major problem during the First World War. See D. S. Linton, "The Obscure Object of Knowledge: German Military Medicine Confronts Gas Gangrene during World War I," *Bulletin of the History of Medicine* 74.2 (2000), 291–316. It was thus a familiar problem by 1954, including cases caused by injections.

26. These were candle-type filters, in which water was filtered by a vertical, stone-like, porous core that was known to be fragile.

27. Cauvin, "Rapport du chef," 7.

28. Ibid., 7–8, for all quotations in this paragraph.

29. Ann L. Stoler, "In Cold Blood: Hierarchies of Credibility and the Politics of Colonial Narratives," *Representations* 37 (1992), 151–89.

30. All quotations in this paragraph are from Cauvin, "Rapport du chef," 6.

31. Christol, "Rapport de l'inspecteur," 4.

32. Ibid.

33. Ibid., 5.

34. Jardin, "Compte rendu du commandant de section de gendarmerie," 2.

35. "Extrait du rapport politique mensuel."

36. Christol, "Rapport de l'inspecteur," 3.

37. Ibid., 5.

38. Gilbrin, "Rapport du chef de région," 7.

39. Christol, "Rapport de l'inspecteur," 6.

40. Gilbrin, "Rapport du chef de région," 7.

41. Christol, "Rapport de l'inspecteur," 5.

42. "Extrait du rapport politique mensuel," 2.

43. Christol, "Rapport de l'inspecteur," 6.

44. Cauvin, "Rapport du chef," 9. The campaigns were suspended immediately following the announcement of the events at Yokadouma while waiting for the results of the investigations.

45. Christol, "Rapport de l'inspecteur," 6.

46. Ibid.

47. "Extrait du rapport politique mensuel."

48. Christol, "Rapport de l'inspecteur," 3–6, for all the following quotations in this paragraph.

49. Bruno Latour, *Reassembling the Social: An Introduction to Actor-Network-Theory* (Oxford University Press, Oxford, 2005).

50. Paule Constant, *C'est fort la France!* (Gallimard, Paris, 2013), 200.

51. Ibid., 201.

52. Ibid., 150.

CHAPTER 8: "We Cried without Making a Palaver"

1. ANY, 3 AC 1871, Christol, "Rapport de l'inspecteur des Affaires administratives du centre. Décès à la suite de la campagne de lomidinisation du GM 15 du SHMP à Yokadouma du 14 au 17 novembre," November 22, 1954, 5.

2. Ibid.

3. ANY, 3 AC 1871, Gilbrin, "Rapport du chef de région de la Boumba-Ngoko à M. le haut-commissaire de la République française au Cameroun. Accidents mortels suite passage GMT 15," November 19, 1954, 7.

4. This is based on the definitions suggested in Luc Boltanski et al. (eds.), *Affaires, scandales et grandes causes. De Socrate à Pinochet* (Stock, Paris, 2007), 14. Although the colonial issue is not addressed in this collection, numerous scandals linked to colonial Africa animated metropolitan France, from the Voulet-Chanoine affair to that of the Congo-Ocean railway. See Bertrand Taithe, *The Killer Trail: A Colonial Scandal in the Heart of Africa* (Oxford University Press, Oxford, 2009).

5. Damien de Blic and Cyril Lemieux, "Le scandale comme épreuve. Éléments de sociologie pragmatique," *Politix* 71 (2005), 9–38, 14–15.

6. Boltanski et al., *Affaires, scandales et grandes causes*, 8.

7. Blic and Lemieux, "Le scandale comme épreuve," 11–13.

8. Ann L. Stoler, "Colonial Archives and the Arts of Governance," *Archival Science* 2.1–2 (2002), 87–109.

9. Ann L. Stoler, "Colonial Archives and the Arts of Governance: On the Content of the Form," in C. Hamilton et al. (eds.), *Refiguring the Archive* (Kluwer Academic, Dordrecht, 2002), 83–102, 92.

10. Louis-Ferdinand Céline, *L'église* (Denoël et Steele, Paris, 1933), 45–46.

11. ANY, 3 AC 1871, Haut-Commissariat de la république, "Notes manuscrites," December 28, 1954.

12. Richard A. Joseph, *Radical Nationalism in Cameroon: Social Origins of the U.P.C. Rebellion* (Clarendon, Oxford, 1977); Achille Mbembe, *La naissance du maquis dans le Sud Cameroun,*

1920–1960 (Karthala, Paris, 1996); Thomas Deltombe, Manuel Domergue, and Jacob Tatsitsa, *Kamerun! Une guerre cachée aux origines de la Françafrique, 1948–1971* (La Découverte, Paris, 2011).

13. Haut-Commissariat de la république, "Notes manuscrites."

14. Gilbrin, "Rapport du chef de région de la Boumba-Ngoko," 3.

15. ANY, 3 AC 1871, "Télégramme officiel chiffré de région Yokadouma pour haut-commissaire de la RF au Cameroun, no. 11," November 16, 1954.

16. ANY, 3 AC 1871, "Télégramme officiel chiffré de haut-commissaire de la RF au Cameroun pour région Yokadouma," November 16, 1954.

17. ANY, 3 AC 1871, Assemblée territoriale du Cameroun, "Session budgétaire d'octobre 1954. PV de la séance plénière du 15 novembre 1954," 9–10.

18. Janvier Onana, *Le sacre des indigènes évolués. Essai sur la professionnalisation politique (L'exemple du Cameroun)* (Dianoïa, Chennevières-sur-Marne, France, 2004).

19. Jean-François Bayart, *L'état au Cameroun* (Presses de la Fondation Nationale des Sciences Politiques, Paris, 1979), 38–39. Mbida would be elected as a deputy to the National Assembly in Paris before his mentor Louis-Paul Aujoulat and Charles Assalé (two representatives of the health service) in January 1956. Joseph, *Radical Nationalism in Cameroon*, 295–96, 322.

20. Joseph, *Radical Nationalism in Cameroon*, 243–44; Bayart, *L'état au Cameroun*, 23–52.

21. Jacques Ferret, *Les cendres du Manengouba* (L'Harmattan, Paris, 1996), 176–79.

22. Assemblée territoriale du Cameroun, "Session budgétaire d'octobre 1954. PV de la séance plénière du 15 novembre 1954."

23. Ibid.

24. Ibid.

25. ANY, 3 AC 1871, Direction des affaires administratives et politiques, "Rapport confidentiel du haut-commissaire au Ministre de la France d'Outre-Mer. Accidents survenus au cours campagne lomidinisation région Boumba-Ngoko," December 31, 1954.

26. Assemblée territoriale du Cameroun, "Session budgétaire d'octobre 1954. PV de la séance plénière du 15 novembre 1954."

27. "Télégramme officiel chiffré de région Yokadouma pour haut-commissaire de la RF au Cameroun, no. 11."

28. ANY, 3 AC 1871, "Télégramme officiel chiffré de région Yokadouma pour haut-commissaire de la RF au Cameroun, no. 12," November 16, 1954.

29. Jacques Revel, "Micro-analyse et construction du social," in Jacques Revel (ed.), *Jeux d'échelles. La micro-analyse à l'expérience* (Gallimard/Seuil, Paris, 1996), 13–36.

30. ANY, 3 AC 1871, "Télégramme officiel clair de région Yokadouma pour haut-commissaire de la RF au Cameroun, no. 1006/TO/RFN," December 11, 1954; and "Télégramme officiel clair de région Yokadouma pour haut-commissaire de la RF au Cameroun, no. 1027/TO/RFN," December 12, 1954.

31. Christian Bonah and Jean-Paul Gaudillière, "Faute, accident ou risque iatrogène? La régulation des événements indésirables du médicament à l'aune des affaires Stalinon et Distilbène," *Revue Française des Affaires Sociales* 3–4 (2007), 123–51; Sophie Chauveau, *L'invention pharmaceutique. La pharmacie française entre l'état et la société au XXe siècle* (Institut d'Édition Sanofi-Synthélabo, Paris, 1999), 438–44.

32. Guillaume Lachenal, "Franco-African Familiarities: A History of the Pasteur Institute of Cameroon," in Mark Harrison (ed.), *Hospitals beyond the West* (Orient Longman, New Delhi, 2009), 411–44.

33. Félix-Roland Moumié was assassinated in 1960 by the French secret services. Marthe Moumié, his wife, published a personal account that evokes the links between his medical and political work. Marthe Moumié, *Victime du colonialisme français. Mon mari Félix Moumié* (Duboiris, Paris, 2006). Thomas Deltombe and others mention that Félix Moumié was trans-

ferred to Batouri in October 1954. I was not able to verify this (my sources indicate a posting in Maroua until February 1955 and then a transfer to Douala). If Deltombe is correct, Moumié's presence so close to the site of the Lomidinization accident would certainly be a main reason for the administration's concern.

34. Nancy Rose Hunt, *A Nervous State: Violence, Remedies, and Reverie in Colonial Congo* (Duke University Press, Durham, NC, 2016).

35. ANY, 3 AC 1871, "Télégramme officiel chiffré du haut-commissaire de la RF au Cameroun pour France Outre-Mer Paris (nos. 157–58) et Délé France New York (nos. 109–10)," November 19, 1954.

36. AA, 4 485/1067, Ministère des colonies, "Communication au Service de l'hygiène," November 23, 1954.

37. Meredith Terreta, *Nation of Outlaws: State of Violence, Grassfields Tradition, and State Building in Cameroon* (Ohio University Press, Athens, 2014), 3–4.

38. ANY, 3 AC 1871, Assemblée territoriale du Cameroun, "Session extraordinaire d'octobre 1954. PV de la séance plénière du 18 novembre 1954," 12.

39. Ibid., 14.

40. Ibid., 15.

41. Ibid.

42. "Lettre des chefs de canton au haut-commissaire et au procureur général, Yokadouma," November 19, 1954, reprinted in ANY, 3 AC 1871, Gilbrin, "Rapport du chef de région de la Boumba-Ngoko à M. le haut-commissaire de la République française au Cameroun. Accidents mortels suite passage GMT 15," November 19, 1954.

43. ANY, 3 AC 1871, "Télégramme officiel chiffré de région Yokadouma pour haut-commissaire de la RF au Cameroun, novembre 14 à 18," November 18, 1954, with handwritten annotations by the high commissioner.

44. ANY, 3 AC 1871, "Extrait du rapport politique mensuel, région Boumba-Ngoko," February 1955.

45. Jean Mouchet, interview with author, 2003.

46. Personal archives of Alice Botétémé, telegram from the high commissioner to the chief regional officer, December 7, 1954, and Cameroonian Medal of Merit of Théodore Botétémé, December 29, 1954.

47. ANY, 3 AC 1871, "Extrait du rapport politique mensuel, région Boumba-Ngoko," December 1954.

48. Achille Mbembe, "The Power of the Archive and Its Limits," in C. Hamilton et al. (eds.), *Refiguring the Archive* (Kluwer Academic, Boston, 2002), 18–26, 22.

49. ANY, 3 AC 1871, Secrétariat général du haut-commissariat de la République française au Cameroun, "Note pour Monsieur le directeur des affaires politiques et administratives," December 2, 1954.

50. Mbembe, "Power of the Archive," 22.

51. Direction des affaires administratives et politiques, "Rapport confidentiel du haut-commissaire," 3.

CHAPTER 9: The Misfires of the Imperial Machine

1. Paul Farmer, *Pathologies of Power: Health, Human Rights, and the New War on the Poor* (University of California Press, Berkeley, 2003), 144.

2. James E. McClellan and François Regourd, "The Colonial Machine: French Science and Colonization in the Ancien Regime," *Osiris* 15 (2000), 31–50.

3. Ann L. Stoler, *Along the Archival Grain: Epistemic Anxieties and Colonial Common Sense* (Princeton University Press, Princeton, NJ, 2008).

4. Ben Kafka, *Le démon de l'écriture. Pouvoirs et limites de la paperasse* (Zones Sensibles, Brussels, 2013), 17.

5. IMTSSA, box 253, "Télégramme chiffré no. 154 de Afcour Yaoundé à France Outre-Mer Paris," November 17, 1954.

6. For a general overview, see Laurence Monnais-Rousselot, *Médecine et colonisation. L'aventure indochinoise, 1860–1939* (CNRS Éditions, Paris, 1999).

7. Léon Lapeyssonnie, *Toubib des tropiques* (Robert Laffont, Paris, 1982), 130n1.

8. The "4th Office" refers to the directorate of the health service at the Ministry of Overseas France. For example, see IMTSSA, box 253, Gouverneur-général de l'AEF, "Lettre 4205/DGSP-2-HC, au secrétaire d'etat à la France d'Outre-Mer," December 31, 1954.

9. Pierre Bourdieu, Olivier Christin, and Pierre Étienne Will, "Sur la science de l'état," *Actes de la Recherche en Sciences Sociales* 133 (2000), 3–9, 5.

10. Ann L. Stoler, "Colonial Archives and the Arts of Governance," *Archival Science* 2.1–2 (2002), 103.

11. Handwritten annotation on "Télégramme chiffré no. 154."

12. ANY, 3 AC 1871, Haut-Commissariat de la république, "Notes manuscrites," December 28, 1954.

13. IMTSSA, box 253, Ministère de la santé et de la population, Service central de la pharmacie, "Lettre au Ministre de la France d'Outre-Mer, Direction du Service de santé," November 19, 1954.

14. Stoler, *Along the Archival Grain*, 25–28.

15. IMTSSA, box 253, Dr. de Marqueissac, "Présentation—Conditionnement et prix de la Lomidine," December 1, 1954, 1–2.

16. IMTSSA, box 253, "Télégramme clair no. 70129 de France-Outremer à hauts-commissaires AOF, AEF, Cameroun, et commissaire Togo," December 3, 1954.

17. IMTSSA, box 253, Médecin-général Robert, "Lettre aux hauts-commissaires de la république en AOF, en AEF et au Cameroun et au commissaire de la république au Togo," December 14, 1954, 2.

18. IMTSSA, box 253, Gouverneur-général de l'AEF, "Lettre no. 4147/DGSP-2–HC au secrétaire d'état à la France d'Outre-Mer," December 27, 1954, 1–2; and Médecin-général Talec, "Lettre au médecin-général inspecteur," February 18, 1954.

19. Arch. Spécia, box 124, 8313626B124, Direction commerciale, "Lettre à Direction technique, Spécia St-Fons et Direction générale," December 6, 1954.

20. Arch. Spécia, box 124, 8313626B124, Spécia Saint-Fons, "Lettre à Direction technique," December 8, 1954.

21. IMTSSA, box 101, Médecin-général Cheneveau, "Rapport annuel. Année 1954. Commentaires," 113–14.

22. ANY, 3 AC 1871, "Télégramme officiel chiffré de région Batouri pour haut-commissaire de la RF au Cameroun, no. 22," November 22, 1954, annotated.

23. The quotations in the following paragraphs are drawn from IMTSSA, box 253, André Lotte, "Rapport complémentaire sur les accidents sur les accidents septiques observés dans le secteur IV," March 4, 1953; and Gouverneur-général de l'AEF, "Lettre no. 72 DGSP à Monsieur le secrétaire d'état de la France d'Outre-Mer," January 12, 1953.

24. Lotte, "Rapport complémentaire," 4.

25. IMTSSA, box 253, Médecin-colonel Lavergne, "Lettre du 26 décembre 1952 au procureur de la république [copie]," January 31, 1953.

26. P. W. Harvey and G. V. Purnell, "Fatal Case of Gas Gangrene Associated with Intramuscular Injections," *British Medical Journal* 1.5594 (1968), 744–46.

27. Lavergne, "Lettre du 26 décembre 1952."

28. Gaston Muraz, "Oui, l'Afrique intertropicale peut et doit guérir de la maladie du sommeil en généralisant la lomidinisation de toutes ses régions contaminées," *L'Essor Médical dans l'Union Française* 3 (1954), 24.

29. Médecin-colonel Richet, "Quelques considérations sur la chimio-prophylaxie de la trypanosomiase humaine en A.E.F.," in *International Scientific Committee for Trypanosomiasis Research: Fifth Meeting, Held at Pretoria 13th to 17th September, 1954* (BPITT, Léopoldville, 1954), 76.

30. Ibid. Accidents similar to those in Yokadouma and Nkoltang were reported in Saa in Cameroon around 1953–54, in Nola in Oubangui-Chari in 1953 (cited by Muraz, "Oui, l'Afrique intertropicale"), and in another sector in French Equatorial Africa by F. Gauthier, *Lutte contre la trypanosomiase et la lèpre en Afrique 1953–1960. Mission d'une équipe médicale mobile de prospection du Service général d'hygiène et de prophylaxie* (Éditions des Écrivains, Paris, 2000).

31. Arch. Spécia, box 124, 8313626B124, Jacques Pierre Ziegler, letter to Dr. de Marqueissac, reproduced in "Lettre de la Direction technique, no. 2703," June 25, 1953, from which the following quotations are also drawn.

32. Ibid.

33. Ibid. Dr. Mainette has not been identified.

34. Ibid.

35. Direction commerciale, "Lettre à Direction technique."

36. ANY, 3 AC 1871, Le procureur général près la Cour d'appel, "Lettre no. 644/CF/CO au haut-commissaire de la République française au Cameroun," July 7, 1956, from which quotations below are also drawn.

37. ANY, 3 AC 1871, Médecin-lieutenant-colonel Cauvin, "Rapport du chef du Service d'hygiène mobile et de prophylaxie à monsieur le directeur des services de la Santé publique au Cameroun," November 24, 1954, 7.

38. Le procureur général, "Lettre no. 644/CF/CO."

39. Ibid.

40. Michel Foucault, "Crise de la médecine ou de l'anti-médecine?" in his *Dits et écrits, 1954–1988*, vol. 2 (Gallimard, Paris, 1994), 40–58.

41. "Mobile hygiene is economical and, as long as it is rational, profitable, this is a reason for maintaining at all costs an action on which depends, definitively, the very survival of these impoverished regions." IMTSSA, box 253, André Lotte, "La prophylaxie de la maladie du sommeil dans les zones aquatiques."

42. Jean Mouchet, interview with author, 2003.

43. Letter from the canton chiefs to the high commissioner and to the attorney general, Yokadouma, November 19, 1954, cited in Gilbrin, "Rapport du chef de région de la Boumba-Ngoko à M. le haut-commissaire de la République française au Cameroun. Accidents mortels suite passage GMT 15," November 19, 1954.

44. Muraz, "Oui, l'Afrique intertropicale," 24, emphasis in original.

45. Cauvin, "Rapport du chef," 9.

46. IMTSSA, box 110, Médecin-colonel Vaisseau, "Rapport annuel. Année 1948. Service de la Santé publique. Cameroun français," 114.

47. Jean Mouchet, interview with author, 2003.

48. Ibid.

CHAPTER 10: The Swan Song of Eradication

1. AA, 4485/1067, Dr. G. Neujean, "Chimiothérapie et chimioprophylaxie de la maladie du sommeil à *T. gambiense*. Rapport présenté au 6e Congrès international de médecine tropicale," Lisbon, September 5–13, 1958, 9–10 (emphasis in original).

2. Académie royale des sciences d'Outre-Mer and P. Janssens, "Neujean," in *Biographie belge d'Outre-Mer*, vol. 8 (Académie Royale des Sciences d'Outre-Mer, Brussels, 1998), 317–24. Georges Neujean (1907–72) worked in Congo from the 1930s and directed the Princess Astrid Institute of Tropical Medicine in Léopoldville.

3. IMTSSA, box 249, Jean Demarchi, "Rapport sur la chimioprophylaxie de la trypanosom-iase à *T. gambiense*."

4. IMTSSA, box 112, "Service de santé publique, année 1957," 59.

5. Demarchi, "Rapport sur la chimioprophylaxie."

6. Bib. IMTA, Direction générale des services médicaux—Congo belge, "Rapport annuel 1955," 62–64; and Direction générale des services médicaux—Congo belge, "Rapport annuel 1957," 54–56.

7. PAM stands for penicillin aluminum monostearate. The method and its use in mobile campaigns were developed in Haiti for the yaws eradication program lauched by the WHO and UNICEF from the 1950s. The strategy aimed to treat both people who tested positive and their "contacts," who might be healthy carriers. But screening was quickly identified as its most expensive step, and the total treatment of populations appeared to be the most cost-effective solution. David McBride, *Missions for Science: US Technology and Medicine in America's African World* (Rutgers University Press, New Brunswick, NJ, 2002), 201–5.

8. "Report of Second International Conference on Control of Yaws, Nigeria, 1955: II," *Journal of Tropical Medicine and Hygiene* 60.3 (1957), 62–73.

9. C. J. Hackett and C. W. Gockel, "Equipment and Technique of Intramuscular Injection in Mass Treatment Campaigns against the Treponematoses," *Bulletin of the World Health Organization* 19.3 (1958), 531–45, 541.

10. IMTSSA, box 249, documents of the Comité scientifique international pour les recherches sur la trypanosomiase, 1954–58.

11. The Organisation de coordination et de coopération pour la lutte contre les grandes endémies (Organization for Coordination and Cooperation in the Control of Major Endemic Diseases) was created in 1961, and the Organisation de coordination pour la lutte contre les endémies en Afrique centrale (Organization for Coordination of Control of Endemic Diseases in Central Africa) was created in 1962 on the model of the first, initially under the name of OCCGEAC (Organisation de coordination et de coopération pour la lutte contre les grandes endémies en Afrique centrale; Organization for Coordination and Cooperation in the Control of Major Endemic Diseases in Central Africa). The creation of the OCCGE is described by P. Richet, "L'histoire et l'œuvre de l'OCCGE en Afrique occidentale francophone," *Transactions of the Royal Society of Tropical Medicine and Hygiene* 59 (1965), 234–54.

12. Guillaume Lachenal, "Célébrer le passé, construire le futur. L'indépendance et le microcosme médical au Cameroun," in Didier Nativel, Odile Goerg, and Farina Rajanoah (eds.), *Les indépendances en Afrique. L'événement et ses mémoires 1957/1960–2010* (Presses Universitaires de Rennes, Rennes, France, 2013), 353–76.

13. M. Vaucel, "La participation française aux activités de santé publique en Afrique francophone et son avenir," *Bulletin de l'Académie Nationale de Médecine* 148 (1964), 232–36; M. Vaucel, "Le service de santé des troupes de marine et la médecine tropicale française," *Transactions of the Royal Society of Tropical Medicine and Hygiene* 59 (1965), 226–33. The colonial corps was renamed Troupes d'Outre-Mer (Overseas Corps), then Troupes de marine (Marine Corps).

14. [Organisation mondiale de la santé], "Introduction," *Bulletin of the World Health Organization* 28 (1963), 537–43, 540.

15. Jean Schneider, "Traitement de la trypanosomiase africaine humaine," *Bulletin of the World Health Organization* 28 (1963), 763–86, 768, 783.

16. Jaime L. Neves, "A prevenção da doença do sono," *Anais da Escola Nacional de Saúde Pública e Medicina Tropical* (Lisbon) 5.3–4 (1971), 317–24.

17. Demarchi, "Rapport sur la chimioprophylaxie," 17.

18. Schneider, "Traitement de la trypanosomiase," 769.

19. Schneider's work for Spécia is barely mentioned in his obituaries. Dr. Schneider (1911–65), a major figure of Parisian tropical medicine, played a significant role in the experiments with chloroquine that Spécia conducted in North Africa during World War II, and he became involved in the trials of other Spécia products in Africa. He worked as a consultant in the supervision of therapeutic research at Spécia and participated in numerous debates about Lomidine beginning in 1948 (for example, about the cases of gangrene in 1953; see Arch. Spécia, box 124, 8313626B124, "Lettre de la Direction technique, no. 2703," June 25, 1953). G. Lavier, "Jean Schneider [1911–65]," *Presse Médicale* 73 (1965), 1599–600; M. Vaucel, "Jean Schneider [1911–65]," *Bulletin de la Société de Pathologie Exotique* 58.1 (1965), 7–9.

20. IMTSSA, box 101, Médecin-général Cheneveau, "Rapport annuel. Année 1954. Commentaires," 114.

21. Demarchi, "Rapport sur la chimioprophylaxie," 57–58.

22. AIPDak, Bibliothèque CSIRT, "Neuvième réunion, Conakry, 1962," CCTA, publication no. 88, 300.

23. Neujean, "Chimiothérapie et chimioprophylaxie," 11.

CHAPTER 11: **How the Drug Became Useless and Dangerous**

1. "Immuno-diagnostic de la maladie du sommeil," perso.orange.fr/jdtr/beta2m.htm, accessed July 2, 2006.

2. Arch. OCEAC, "Rapport final de la 1re conférence technique de l'OCCGEAC, Yaoundé," December 7–11, 1965. The following quotations are from Jean Dutertre's presentation and the ensuing discussion on 505–7.

3. Ibid.

4. Ibid.

5. All the quotations that follow are from Arch. OCEAC, "Rapport final de la IIe conférence technique de l'OCCGEAC, Yaoundé," 1967, 299–305.

6. Ibid.

7. Ibid.

8. Jean-Pierre Dozon, "Quatre modèles de prévention," in Jean-Pierre Dozon and Didier Fassin (eds.), *Critique de la santé publique. Une approche anthropologique* (Balland, Paris, 2001), 23–46.

9. This expression was used with reference to yellow fever prophylaxis. See AIPDak, dir. 1, Médecin-général Durieux, letter to Noël Bernard, March 17, 1952, 4.

10. René Labusquière and Jean Dutertre, "La lutte contre les derniers foyers de trypanosomiase humaine africaine," *Médecine Tropicale* 26.4 (March 1966), 357–62.

11. Manuel G. Correia, "Relatorio do chef da missao de combate as tripanossomiases na Guiné referente ao ano de 1972," *Boletim Cultural da Guiné Portuguesa* 27.108 (1972), 677–749.

12. Marc Wéry, interview with author, 2008.

13. D. Kayembe and M. Wéry, "Observations sur la sensibilité aux diamidines de souches de *Trypanosoma gambiense* récemment isolées en république du Zaire," *Annales de Société Belge de Médecine Tropicale* 52.1 (1972), 1–8, 3–4.

14. Ibid., 6–7.

15. Donatien Kayembe, interview with author, 2007.

16. J.-H. Ricosse et al., "L'épidémiologie actuelle de la trypanosomiase humaine africaine et les problèmes qu'elle pose," *Médecine d'Afrique Noire* 20.4 (1973), 291–300. This aspect, as well as that of cryptic infections, has not been well elucidated retrospectively.

17. Jean Dutertre, "Trypanosomose humaine africaine" (1993, updated in 2003), perso. orange.fr/jdtr/trypoiti.htm, accessed July 22, 2006.

18. IMTSSA, Fonds Richet, box 428, Médecin-général Richet, "Notes manuscrites."

19. Christian Burri and Reto Brun, "Human African Trypanosomiasis," in Gordon C. Cook and Alimuddin I. Zumla (eds.), *Manson's Tropical Diseases*, 21st ed. (Saunders, Philadelphia, 2003), 1303–23, 1321.

20. René Labusquière, *Santé rurale et médecine préventive en Afrique. Stratégie à opposer aux principales affections* (Imprimerie Saint-Paul, Bar-le-Duc, France, 1974), 260.

21. Léon Launoy, "Instruire l'autochtone," *Annales Coloniales Quotidiennes* (August 4, 1928).

22. ANY, 3 AC 1620, Direction des affaires politiques et administratives, "Lettre au gouverneur de l'Oubangui-Chari, Bangui (AEF)," February 12, 1957.

23. Ibid.

Epilogue

1. The site has since been renamed; see londoneast-uk.com, accessed May 30, 2016.

2. John Phillips, "Mini Silicon Valley Planned at Sanofi Site in Dagenham," *Barking and Dagenham Post*, October 17, 2012, http://www.barkinganddagenhampost.co.uk/news/business/mini_silicon_valley_planned_at_sanofi_site_in_dagenham_1_1657730, accessed January 4, 2017.

3. J. E. Lesch, "The Discovery of M&B 693 (Sulfapyridine)," in Gregory Higby and Elaine Condouris Stroud (eds.), *The Inside Story of Medicines: A Symposium* (American Institute of the History of Pharmacy, Madison, WI, 1997), 101–19.

4. For a complete account, see Peter S. Arno and Karyn Feiden, *Against the Odds: The Story of AIDS Drug Development, Politics, and Profits* (HarperCollins, New York, 1992). For a review of PCP prophylaxis, see Pierre-Marie Girard, "Cotrimoxazole ou aérosols de pentamidine dans la prévention de la pneumocystose. L'épreuve des faits," pistes.fr/transcriptases/14_701.htm, accessed July 30, 2013.

5. Randy Shilts, *And the Band Played On: Politics, People, and the AIDS Epidemic* (St. Martin's, New York, 1987), 54, 61, 66; Elizabeth W. Etheridge, *Sentinel for Health: A History of the Centers for Disease Control* (University of California Press, Berkeley, 1992), 321–22.

6. Arch. Spécia, box 994053B4, "Coupures de presse."

7. Jim Eigo et al., *FDA Action Handbook* (September 12, 1988), actupny.org/documents/FDAhandbook1.html, accessed September 12, 2013.

8. Steven Epstein, *Histoire du sida*, vol. 1, *Le virus est-il bien la cause du sida*, and vol. 2, *La grande révolte des malades* (Les Empêcheurs de Penser en Rond, Paris, 2001).

9. Jean-Pierre Brard in Assemblée nationale, "Session ordinaire 1995–1996. Première séance du 19 décembre 1995," *Comptes rendus des débats au cours de la Xe législature (1993–1997)* (Assemblée Nationale, Paris, 1997), 23, http://archives.assemblee-nationale.fr/10/cri/1995–1996-ordinaire1/101.pdf, accessed January 5, 2017. I have made similar estimates of the increase in price per gram of pentamidine between 1981 and 1990.

10. Warren E. Leary, "FDA Allows Wider Use of Drug to Prevent Pneumonia in AIDS," *New York Times*, February 7, 1989.

11. An estimate published by Sanofi in 2011 evaluated the donation at $50 million over a longer period (2001–2011). Sanofi, "Accès au médicament" (2011), sanofi.com/Images/29244_Sanofi_Acces_au_Medicament_2011.pdf, accessed September 12, 2013.

Index

Note: Page numbers in *italic* indicate illustrations.